MEASURING QUALITY IMPROVEMENT IN HEALTHCARE

A Guide to Statistical Process Control Applications

Raymond G. Carey, Ph.D.
Robert C. Lloyd, Ph.D.

Most Quality Resources books are available at quantity discounts when purchased in bulk. For more information contact:

Special Sales Department
Quality Resources
A Division of The Kraus Organization Limited
902 Broadway
New York, NY 10010
800-247-8519

Printed in the United States of America

99   98   97   96   95   10   9   8   7   6   5   4   3   2   1

Quality Resources
A Division of The Kraus Organization Limited
902 Broadway
New York, NY 10010
800-247-8519

∞

The paper used in this publication meets the minimum requirements of American National Standard for Information Sciences—Permanence of Paper for Printed Library Materials, ANSI Z39.48–1984.

ISBN 0–527–76293–8

Library of Congress Cataloging-in-Publication Data

Carey, Raymond G.
    Measuring quality improvement in healthcare : a guide to
  statistical process control applications / Raymond G. Carey, Robert
  C. Lloyd.
        p.   cm.
    Includes bibliographical references and index.
    ISBN 0–527–76293–8
    1. Medical care—Quality control—Statistical methods.   2. Health
  facilities—Evaluation—Statistical methods.   I. Lloyd, Robert C.
  II. Title.
  RA399.A1C365   1995
  362.1'068'5—dc20

                                                                          95-5101
                                                                            CIP

To Rita, Mike, and Marc; and
Gwenn, Devon, and Becky

Contents

List of Figures

List of Tables

Foreword

On January 1, 1993, I had the distinct privilege and honor of attending a New Year's Day reception at the home of my friend and colleague, R. Clifton Bailey of the Health Care Financing Administration. In attendance for what would be his last New Year's Day was W. Edwards Deming. At the reception, upon recognizing that a number of us were working in healthcare quality, Deming remarked that healthcare is a system in need of improvement. None of us disagreed. A fascinating discussion ensued. Regrettably, Dr. Deming died on December 20, 1993, at age 93, but his legacy and teachings live on.

Statisticians are very familiar with the concepts of measurement and statistical process control (SPC), and have been applying them in the industry for decades. However, prior to the mid-1980s, measurement and SPC had not been extensively applied in the healthcare setting. Quality measurement and management systems based heavily upon the application of measurement, SPC, and the teachings of Deming and other quality experts, have since been developed in individual hospitals and hospital systems. Although a wide variety of statistical and quality management techniques have been applied, the simpler techniques, such as descriptive measures, graphical displays, control charts, and survey methods have been best received, understood, and used.

Now quality reform has expanded into the managed care world. In particular, performance measurement in managed care is increasingly employing statistical concepts and approaches for quality improvement. Managed care organizations are now increasingly embracing and applying these quantitative methods in quality management.

The healthcare system, as Dr. Deming observed, needs improvement. Real healthcare reform must have quality improvement as its foundation. Comprehensive, systematic quality improvement can only be made using sound methods of measurement and statistical analysis. Although some application of these techniques has already taken place in the healthcare system, it has been far from comprehensive or systematic. Much remains to be done.

Drs. Carey and Lloyd have performed an excellent service for the healthcare quality community by writing *Measuring Quality Improvement in Healthcare*. The practical, down-to-earth orientation of the book makes it accessible to a wide readership from administrative to clinical to support staff. Though it is oriented to a hospital audience, those in non-hospital healthcare settings should also find it useful. Enjoy the book. Use the ideas. Improve healthcare quality.

Randall K. Spoeri, Ph.D.
Assistant Vice President
National Committee for Quality Assurance (NCQA)
Washington, D.C.
and
Chair-Elect, Health Care Division
American Society for Quality Control
December, 1994

Preface

Why another book on "quality"? Numerous books have been written on quality, total quality management (TQM), continuous quality improvement (CQI), team building, leading teams, facilitating teams, and improving processes. There have also been scores of books written by the well-known gurus of CQI, such as W. Edwards Deming, Joseph M. Juran, Philip B. Crosby, and their disciples on statistical process control theory and tools. However, most of the books on quality have been written for the manufacturing arena. Less attention has been given to service industries. Among service industries, healthcare has perhaps received the least attention.

The concepts of CQI did not at first find fertile soil among hospital and healthcare administrators and providers. In the 1980s, most were thinking in terms of "quality assurance" rather than "quality improvement." Quality assurance concentrated on identifying poor providers rather than defective processes. Providers looked to themselves to determine what should be improved rather than to their customers. They struggled with measurement issues. In general, the healthcare field was slow to commit time and resources to understanding CQI theory and tools. When the authors attended a four-day conference by Dr. Deming in Indianapolis in 1990, only about 25 of the approximately 700 people in attendance were from the healthcare industry.

Even after some healthcare leaders began to look seriously at CQI or TQM in the late 1980s, most of the early efforts went into organizing teams. Much less effort was put into measuring the success of teams in improving processes. Indeed, some questioned whether or not it was possible to measure quality improvement.

When purchasers of care and accrediting bodies began to push providers to document quality, a new army of "healthcare quality consultants" sprung up almost overnight. Many of these new consultants came from the manufacturing industry. While most understood the principles of CQI theory, many were less acquainted with the unique problems that healthcare presented. In addition, most healthcare administrators have not been exposed to CQI theory in their graduate training programs. Similarly, most physicians have not received CQI training in medical school. As a result, both administrators and physicians often find it difficult to use CQI tools to measure the success of their efforts.

There is now a growing demand in healthcare to apply the concepts of quality measurement that have been successfully used in industry. Consultants who could present examples of quality measurement from Toyota, General Motors, and Motorola were less successful in explaining how statistical process control techniques could be used to measure improvement in delivering babies, reducing surgical infection rates, and lowering the mortality rates.

Therefore, we have tried to meet what we sensed is a felt need among healthcare administrators and providers, namely, the need to apply statistical process control (SPC) tools to measure the success of efforts to improve healthcare processes and outcomes. Because we are healthcare professionals, we have been able to develop realistic case studies based on actual situations that occur within the healthcare field. The case studies document how SPC techniques can be applied to different types of data: clinical outcome, clinical process, risk management, financial management, and patient satisfaction data. This book does not give a complete explanation of other aspects of CQI that have been adequately covered elsewhere. Nor is this a book on basic statistics, nor on the construction of control charts, nor on the solutions to the specific problems described in the case studies presented in Chapter 6. It is not a book on developing, facilitating, or leading CQI teams. Finally, although the book is based on the theories of Walter A. Shewhart and W. Edwards Deming, it does not explain Deming's "Theory of Profound Knowledge" nor how his ideas are related to other CQI theorists.

Whereas the focus of this book is the set of case studies presented in Chapter 6, we have tried to place the analysis and interpretation of data into the broader CQI effort. Chapter 1 provides a CQI roadmap and asks basic questions about the meaning of quality and for whom we are trying to measure it. Chapters 2 and 3 discuss issues connected with generating data appropriate for analysis with control charts. Chapter 4 discusses variation. How to depict variation? What are the sources of variation? Chapter 5 summarizes basic control chart theory, including how to select the appropriate chart for the data to be analyzed.

Although the first five chapters provide the underpinning for the twelve case studies presented in Chapter 6, we feel that Chapter 6 contains the unique contribution of this book, insofar as it demonstrates how the CQI measurement tools can be applied to healthcare data. Once again, although the emphasis is on statistical thinking, not on solutions to problem situations, Chapter 7 is devoted to describing how improvement strategies can be developed in response to the type of variation identified by control charts.

Chapter 8 discusses the use of surveys in CQI and presents a viewpoint that is somewhat different from the common wisdom on this subject. The content of this chapter stands somewhat apart from the CQI roadmap presented in Chapter 1 and described in Chapters 2 through 7. However, because surveys are used very heavily by healthcare providers, special consideration has been given to the use of survey research in a CQI context.

The task just described is indeed challenging. The invitation to write this book was extended by Quality Resources because of positive feedback they received from those who have attended our national presentations on quality improvement. It is our hope that the publisher's faith in us will be justified and that the healthcare professionals who read this book will find it helpful in their efforts to measure quality.

Raymond G. Carey
Robert C. Lloyd
January 1995

Acknowledgments

The authors wish to acknowledge the assistance of those who directly and indirectly helped them develop the theory and case studies presented in this book. Judith Ryan, Senior Vice President of the Lutheran General Health System (LGHS), and Elizabeth Gordon, Vice President of the LGHS Research and Education Institute provided us with encouragement and support to write this book. LGHS physicians, especially those on the Medical Staff Quality Assurance Committee, discussed data on their clinical processes in a candid manner without defensiveness.

Outside the LGHS community, the authors express their gratitude to the leadership of the American College of Healthcare Executives who fostered our seminar on "How to Measure Quality." We learned from, as well as taught, scores of hospital executives and managers who attended our classes.

The authors are especially grateful to their friend and colleague, Harold Shafter, M.D., who painstakingly reviewed the draft of the book.

Finally, we are grateful to Irene Leung for preparing many of the graphic images in this book, and to Pam Lantz, who helped us prepare the final copy of our manuscript for publication.

1

Planning Your CQI Journey

It is difficult to go through a day without seeing, reading, or hearing something about quality. Our nation seems to be fixated on the concept. In fact, there are so many quality slogans and expressions around us that it is easy to become numb to most of them. For example, can you name the companies or products associated with the following statements?

- The quality goes in before the name goes on!
- We deliver quality!
- It whispers quality!
- The quality leader!
- Dedicated to quality!
- Quality is job one!
- It's a benchmark for quality![1]

---

[1] Just so those of you who tried to identify these statements do not feel like you were left hanging, the product or company associated with each statement follows:
- We deliver quality! (Domino's Pizza)
- The quality goes in before the name goes on! (Zenith Corporation)
- Dedicated to quality! (Century Baby products)
- Quality is job one! (Ford Motor Company)
- It's a benchmark for quality! (Toyota Corolla)
- It whispers quality! (Geo Prism)
- The quality leader! (AMOCO's Ultimate gasoline)

Some of you may be able to identify the company or product right away. Others may say, "I know I've heard that expression before, but I don't remember who said it." Finally, some of you may say, "Who cares! It's just a slogan. All they really want you to do is just buy their product." Whether you recognize these statements as representing the company's personal pledge to you or see them as nothing more than marketing ploys, the simple fact remains—our country is focused more on quality now than it ever has been in its brief history. This focus is so strong that one writer has gone so far as to say that "Quality has become the business strategy of the 80s and 90s" (Pyzdek, 1990: 1).

In some respects, healthcare professionals were late to enter the quality arena. It is true that quality assurance (QA) has been around for decades. But quality improvement (QI), as defined by the principles of continuous quality improvement (CQI) or total quality management (TQM), has not been part of the historical development of the healthcare industry in the United States.

This distinction is highlighted in Figure 1.1. The top part of this figure shows the traditional approach to QA. For any procedure (e.g., C-section deliveries, medication errors, or nosocomial infections), action will be taken only when the process average exceeds a predetermined threshold. In the case of C-sections, for example, if the threshold is 15 percent, nothing would be done to question the process until more than 15 percent of the deliveries, in a given time period, were performed by C-section. Once the threshold was exceeded, however, questions would be asked. When the process average is under the threshold, no questions would be asked. When the threshold is exceeded, there is panic and finger pointing. When the process average is below the threshold, there is complacency.

A QI approach is depicted in the lower half of Figure 1.1. Here it is recognized that the entire output of the process provides the basis for action, not just those occurrences that are deemed unacceptable because they exceeded a specification limit. When a QI approach is taken, there are basically two options for realizing improvement: (1) reduce the variability in the process and/or

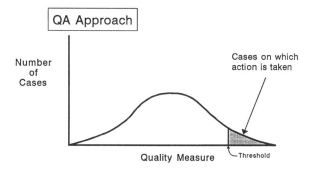

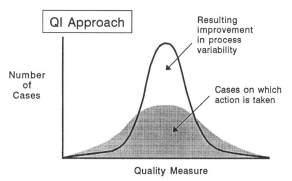

FIGURE 1.1. The difference between quality assurance and quality improvement.

(2) shift the process in the desired direction. Both of these strategies will be discussed in subsequent chapters.

The application and acceptance of a QI perspective in the healthcare industry requires a fundamental shift in the way we view the world in which we work. It requires what the futurist Joel Barker calls a shift in paradigms. Do you see how your job fits into an extended process for the delivery of services and care? Do you think about what happens to the work you perform once you hand it off to the next person? Do you use data to understand how your processes vary over time? Finally, are you more concerned about meeting your budget than modeling behavior that is consistent with the mission, vision, and values of your organization? All of these questions relate to your quality journey. You may not have answers to all of them right now, but if you are serious about QI, you will be confronted by them somewhere along the way.

What Is Quality?

The answer to this question is really quite simple: "It depends!" Although this answer is disturbing to those who want unequivocal answers to complex issues, it is the answer that most quality experts offer to this question. It depends on who are answering the question and what is important to them. It depends on who are defining quality and how they measure it. It depends on the theories you accept to guide your quality journey! If this seems somewhat confusing, do not despair. According to Thomas Pyzdek (1990: Chapter 1), even the quality experts do not agree on a consistent definition of quality. For example, Dr. Joseph Juran's definition of quality revolves around his concept of "fitness for use." His approach is based on the development of interdisciplinary teams that use a variety of diagnostic tools to understand why processes produce products that are not fit for use. Philip Crosby defines quality in terms of performance that produces "zero defects." When defects are produced, it increases the cost of producing quality products or services. For Crosby, producing quality means "conformance to requirements." A third proponent of quality, Dr. W. Edwards Deming, defines quality as a "never-ending cycle of continuous improvement." Deming's system of profound knowledge provides the theoretical basis for his definition. Although these individuals may differ in their definitions of quality, the one element that is common to all three approaches is that management must accept and demonstrate leadership if quality is to be achieved.

Figure 1.2 provides an analogy for the challenge of defining quality. In this picture, there are four blind men who have been asked to describe an elephant. Because they had never encountered an elephant before, all they had to rely on were their senses. One of the blind men touched the elephant's leg. He concluded that the elephant was like a tree because the area he touched was

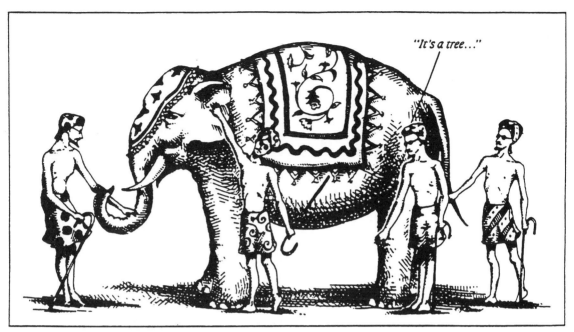

FIGURE 1.2. What is quality?

round, rough, and flared as it entered the ground. The second blind man touched the elephant's tail and concluded that it was like a snake because it was wiggling and round. The third man felt the elephant's trunk and decided that this creature was like a rope because it's surface was bristled and felt as if it were woven. Finally, the last blind man felt the elephant's side and said that the elephant was like a large wall because he could not find the beginning or the end of the creature. The point is that they are all right and yet they are all wrong! Their perceptions of an elephant were based on their individual perspectives and experience. In many ways, the same problem occurs when defining quality. We define it as we see it, and as it has meaning to our frame of reference. Rarely do we think about quality as others perceive it.

In the healthcare industry, quality has been historically defined by those who provide care. Since the early 1980s, however, there has been a growing desire on the part of customers to decide for themselves the meaning of quality. For example, during the mid-1980s, business coalitions, purchaser groups, and lobbying organizations entered the growing debate over the cost and quality of healthcare. These groups pushed for the public release of data documenting the quality of care provided by physicians and hospitals. It was also during this time period that state data commissions became very popular sources for tracking the "cost and quality" of provider services.

In spite of many initiatives, such as those sponsored by the Joint Commission on Accreditation of Healthcare Organizations (JCAHO) and the National Committee on Quality Assurance (NCQA), it appears that purchasers and providers have been unable to arrive at consensus on a uniform definition of quality. What is apparent is that if providers wish to maintain leadership in defining quality, they need to (1) become active participants in the public debate over quality; (2) take a close look at the ways in which they have been defining quality; (3) ask themselves if their definitions are aligned with what the purchasers of care define as being important; (4) develop meaningful measures of quality and data collection systems that allow them to demonstrate quality and value; and (5) be willing to share data not only on aggregated outcomes, but also on measures that are specific to individual procedures, service lines, and/or groups of physicians.

Who Is Interested in Quality?

There was a time when the quality assurance (QA) committees of hospitals were the primary bodies interested in documenting the quality of healthcare services. During this era, data were closely guarded and the only external people who gained access to hospital data were lawyers who were collecting depositions or preparing for malpractice suits. Today, the game has changed—data on quality, costs, charges, payments, patient satisfaction, and outcomes are of key interest to many groups and individuals. Gone are the days when only the QA committee looked at the hospital's quality data. General consensus seems to be that data should be shared with the consumers of healthcare. What remains unclear, however, is the level of detail that should be shared and how consumers will use provider-based data to actually make informed decisions about quality.

There are two basic categories of customers interested in measuring quality. First, there are **internal customers,** such as the board of directors, individual physicians and other clinicians, as well as healthcare managers and employees. Each of these groups needs to measure or evaluate quality for different reasons. They also have different demands for detail, the frequency of collecting data, and how quickly they receive results. For example, clinicians need to have detailed data that are provided in a fairly short time period. Typically, this is procedure or testing data that help the clinicians make decisions about the care being delivered to an individual patient. Hospital managers, on the other hand, may not need to have patient-specific data. They may decide that aggregated data that summarize the total volume of procedures, average turnaround times for tests, and total costs for a particular group of patients are sufficient for their needs.

External customers comprise the second group of individuals who are interested in measuring healthcare quality. Within this category are patients and their care givers, private and public purchasers/payer groups, accrediting/regulatory agencies, academic institutions/researchers, and the media. The diversity of these groups and the factors that motivate them to seek quality data have created a whole new set of pressures for providers. The extent of these demands has been documented in *Inventory of External Data Demands Placed on Hospitals*, published by the Hospital Research and Educational Trust (1990). On occasion, some of these external groups have pursued access to quality data for political purposes. At other times, external customers have had a more objective interest in quality data so they could make more informed healthcare choices or conduct academic research. Regardless of the reason for the request, the simple fact remains that interest in quality data by external customers has grown dramatically.

Confronted with these new demands, providers are challenged to gain new insights about customer wants and expectations. Without listening to the voice of the customer, providers will be unable to know whether the processes they have in place are capable of meeting the expectations of the customers. An imbalance between what the customer expects (the voice of the customer) and what the process is capable of producing (the voice of the process) will inevitably lead to customer defections, decreases in quality, increased costs, and wasted effort. Therefore, the role of management in all of this is to bring the voice of the process into alignment with the voice of the customer. Although all of this may sound a little overwhelming, there are a number of tools and techniques, described in this book that can be used to address the complexity of meeting customer expectations, improve the output of our healthcare system, and reduce waste and rework. Before applying the tools and techniques to a specific quality improvement initiative, however, it is useful to have a quality improvement roadmap to guide your journey.

A Quality Improvement Road Map

There is an old expression that maintains that a journey of a thousand miles must begin with a single step. Your quality improvement journey needs to begin at a point that will start you off on the correct foot. Unfortunately, not every team thinks about where it wishes to be in the future and starts by developing solutions to a perceived problem before it has clearly defined the problem and its boundaries. If you are not sure of your direction, any path will take you there. The ideas presented in this book are not based on a random walk toward improvement. They are based on a well-tested roadmap that is presented in Figure 1.3.

Figure 1.3 not only provides a road map for improving a process, but it also serves as the basic outline for the remainder of this book. Subsequent chapters provide additional detail on each of the steps in this flowchart. Because this book deals primarily with using control charts to analyze and interpret healthcare data,

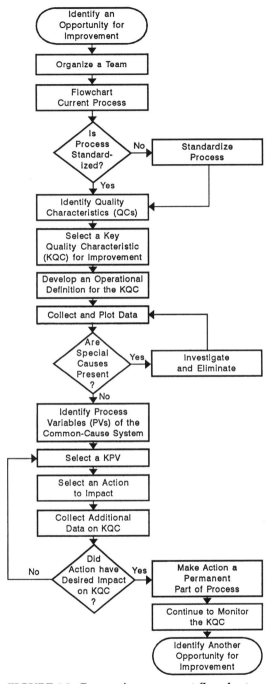

FIGURE 1.3. Process improvement flowchart.

however, more attention is given to those steps that address data collection, understanding variation in the process, and detecting special causes. Although this roadmap may appear to be very structured, it provides sufficient latitude that teams can add their own unique interpretations once they have a firm grasp of the diagram's major principles.

The journey begins by **identifying an opportunity for improvement.** This may come from listening to the voice of the customer, for example, by conducting needs assessments, by collecting survey results, by observation, or by listening to customer complaints. Out of the many opportunities available, you will have to be specific about what your team will and will not be doing. Everyone should have a common perspective on where the process begins and ends.

Once an opportunity is identified, the next task is to **organize a team.** Your team should have representatives from all areas involved with the improvement opportunity. For example, if your team is trying to improve the scheduling process in Family Practice, you would want to have all participants in the process represented on the team. This might include clerical personnel who schedule appointments, nurses, physicians, and the practice manager. Inviting only physicians and administrators to be on such a team will greatly limit the team's ability to understand the process and will negate the support needed by those who actually do the scheduling.

Developing a flowchart of the current process is among the first tasks before the team. Note that this is not a flowchart for the ideal process or one that you think should be in place. Your ability to improve a process will depend on how well you understand the current process and how well your flowchart represents reality. As a result of developing your flowchart, you should be in a position to ask whether the process is standardized. If you determine that the process is done in six different ways, it will be almost impossible to improve the process because you do not have one process. You have six! For example, if your hospital sends specimens to the lab by the pneumatic tube system, by lab techs who make periodic rounds, and by unit secretaries who make special trips to deliver specimens, you do not have a standardized process. Before you proceed on your journey, your team should work to **agree on one standardized process** for delivering specimens. If you do not take time to accomplish this standardization, how will you know which process you are trying to improve?[2]

The next step is to **identify the customers** of the process. You might initially identify several customers. Deciding on the primary customer is essential, however, before you can identify what the customer perceives to be important.

Those aspects of the process which the primary customer identifies as important are called **quality characteristics** (QCs). The challenge of the team is to sort through the QCs and decide which one will be the **key quality characteristic** (KQC). The KQC will be the focal point of the team's efforts.

Once the KQC is selected, the team is ready to move on to **development of an operational definition** of the KQC and the **development of a data collection plan.** When data have been collected, a run or control chart can be made and the next question can be addressed (i.e., Are there special causes of variation present in the process?). If special causes are detected, then the team must work to eliminate the special causes from the process; otherwise, they will continue to make the process unpredictable and "out of control." When the process is exhibiting only common-cause variation, the team is ready to start developing an improvement strategy.

The steps in the development of an improvement strategy are also sequential and begin with **identifying process variables (PVs).** These are the variables thought to have the greatest impact on the KQC. From the list of all potential PVs, **one key process variable (KPV)** should be selected and an improvement strategy

---

[2]There may be occasions when a process has deteriorated to the point that it has to be completely redesigned, rather than standardized. In these instances, the team should alter its intent from quality improvement to process reengineering. The focus of this book is process improvement. Readers who wish more information on process reengineering may find help from a variety of resources, for example, Roberts (1994) and the September 1994 issue of the *Quality Letter*.

should be developed around this variable. An **action related to the KPV** is then implemented, more data are collected, and the impact of the KPV on the KQC is evaluated. After implementing its improvement strategy, the team needs to determine whether the selected action had the desired impact. If it did not have the desired impact, then another KPV should be selected and its impact evaluated. If, on the other hand, the action appears to have improved the process, then steps should be taken to make the action a permanent part of the process.

Finally, there is a need to establish a mechanism to **monitor the process** on an ongoing basis. This ensures that the observed improvements are maintained and that the process does not slip back to its initial level of unacceptable performance. This ongoing monitoring may be done at a less intense level than when you were trying to determine whether special causes were present. After a process for ongoing monitoring is in place, another opportunity for improvement would be identified and the journey would be started again.

2

Preparing to Collect Data

All too often, people are more interested in making and interpreting run or control charts than they are with thinking about all of the steps that lead to the successful use of the charts. Yet without adequate preparation, the results of your efforts will be generally unacceptable. This conclusion should not be foreign to the reader. There are many parallels in everyday life. For example, readers who have tried to paint their own home will undoubtedly recall that the actual painting of your home was the easiest part of the process. Preparing your house to be painted, however, required much more time and effort than the actual painting. Perhaps you needed to scrape away the old paint, sand the uneven spots, and fill in holes in the wood. You took care with these preparations, so that the new coat of paint would look nice and last a long time. In the same way, constructing and interpreting a run or control chart will be much easier if you have prepared properly. Before starting to collect data, therefore, it is recommended that seven preparatory quality improvement steps be considered. These steps are reflected in the CQI road map presented at the end of the last chapter.

Identifying an Opportunity for Improvement

Your first task is to identify an opportunity for improvement. Which processes are you going to improve? Which one will you initiate first? How you approach answering these questions depends on your work area and your responsibilities within your area. For example, are your primary customers internal (e.g., physicians or other managers) or are your customers external (e.g., patients, businesses, or managed care organizations)? As you are aware by now, the key to identifying an appropriate opportunity for improvement is to do so from your customer's point of view rather than from your own. Listening to customer complaints and simply observing your processes are the obvious ways to begin to look for an opportunity to improve.

If time and resources are available, focus groups provide an excellent way to listen to the voice of the customer. To conduct a focus group, you identify a small number of your customers, invite them to sit down with you for an hour or two to discuss issues that they feel are important and the extent to which they feel these issues are being addressed. Focus groups have the advantage of allowing you to probe issues and concerns at some length. However, focus groups have the disadvantage of not allowing you to generalize your findings to the entire customer population. For example, if 8 out of 10 patients in a given focus group report that they were not pleased with the nurses' response times to the call buttons during their last hospital stay, you have no way of knowing whether this percentage is representative of all patients. (A more complete discussion of focus groups can be found in M. Q. Patton, *How to Use Qualitative Methods in Evaluation*, 1987.)

Surveys can also be an excellent tool for identifying and prioritizing opportunities for improvement, but only if they are executed carefully and professionally. Although well-conducted surveys allow you to generalize your findings to your entire group of customers, surveys usually require more time and money to execute than focus groups. Because of the potentially great value of survey research in measuring the voice of the customer, the use of surveys for CQI is discussed in greater detail in Chapter 8.

For those who are looking for other ways to identify improvement opportunities, Sloan (1994) has suggested over 100 possible CQI projects in 20 different service areas of healthcare facilities.

For example, those involved in alcohol and drug programs might look at recidivism rate or the medication cost per patient. Those in emergency services might investigate waiting time to see a physician or patients leaving against medical advice. Medical records personnel might investigate delinquent medical records, the number of charting errors, or transcription turnaround time. Although many of Sloan's suggestions focus on reducing cost, his ideas can serve as a starting point for identifying other opportunities for improvement.

Other suggestions are provided by Dr. Donald Berwick (1993) who identified four general areas in which changes in processes might lead to improved healthcare delivery:

1. Health status outcomes

2. The experience of care

3. The total cost of care and illness

4. Social justice and equity in health

Within the first category, Berwick suggests four ways to improve health status outcomes: (1) increasing appropriateness of practice (by reducing the use of inappropriate surgery, admissions, and tests); (2) increasing effective preventive practice (by reducing causes of illness such as smoking, hand-gun violence, and alcohol and cocaine abuse); (3) reducing cesarean-section rates without compromise in maternal or fetal outcomes; and (4) streamlining pharmaceutical use, especially for antibiotics and drug prescriptions for the elderly. Next, he suggests that we might find opportunities to improve the experience of care by increasing the frequency with which patients participate actively in decision making about therapeutic options, and by decreasing waiting in all its forms. Third, he suggested reducing the total cost of care by consolidating high-technology services into regional and community-wide centers by reducing wasteful and duplicate recording, and by reducing inventory levels. Finally, he suggested improving social justice and equity in healthcare by reducing the difference between the black and white populations in infant mortality and low birth weight.

Prioritizing Opportunities

Regardless of the method by which you choose to listen to the voice of your customer, you will undoubtedly identify more possible opportunities for improving your process than you have time and resources to address. Therefore, you must narrow down your opportunities to what is manageable and what will provide the best return on your efforts. One way to approach the question, "On which problem should we concentrate our efforts?" is to use a Pareto analysis. The Pareto analysis was named after a nineteenth-century Italian economist (Vilfredo Pareto), who observed that a small minority of people in Italy owned the greater proportion of land and means of production. His work led him to the conclusion that 20 percent of the people in Italy owned 80 percent of the wealth.

Dr. Joseph Juran applied the Pareto principle to CQI theory for the purpose of determining which of many potential opportunities should be pursued first. Pareto analysis is the process of ranking opportunities to determine which of many potential opportunities should be pursued first. It is also known as "separating the vital few from the trivial many," because for any groups of things that contribute to a common effect, a relatively few contributors account for a majority of the effect. For an extended discussion of Pareto charts, see Plsek and Onnias (1989).

Pareto analysis should be used at various stages in a quality improvement program to determine which step to take next. It is used to answer such questions as "Which KQC should we address first?" and "On what type of problem should we concentrate our efforts?" A Pareto diagram will direct your attention to the most frequent defects or nonconformaties, but not necessarily the most important ones.

Many computer software programs allow you to do a Pareto analysis with great ease. For example, Figure 2.1 shows how Pareto

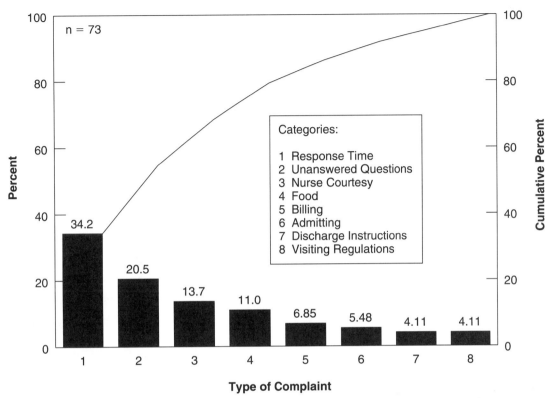

FIGURE 2.1. Pareto diagram of patient complaints (tabulated from write-in comments in a recent patient survey).

analysis was used to prioritize patient complaints and to identify which opportunities for improvement might be pursued first. The figure shows the results of tabulation of write-in comments from a patient survey. Of 73 written complaints, 34.2 percent were concerned with "nurse response time," that is, patients complaining that their call buttons were not answered promptly. 20.5 percent complained that their questions were not answered to their satisfaction, and another 13.7 percent complained about "nursing courtesy." Together, these three complaint categories accounted for approximately 70 percent of all write-in complaints (i.e., the vital few). Although other patients complained about the food, admitting and billing procedures, inadequacy of discharge instructions, and visiting regulations, these latter complaints accounted for less than one-third of all patient write-in comments and can be considered the "common many." Therefore, given these data, a CQI team that wished to address improving patient relations would do well to focus on the three most common complaints that together amounted to over two-thirds of the complaints.

Organizing a Team

Once an opportunity for improvement has been selected, you ought to ask whether or not you can address it by yourself or whether you need a team. There are some problems with your process that you might consider addressing by yourself or with another coworker. However, for more complex processes, more than one person may be needed. A team is more likely than a single individual to consider all aspects of a problem and to have more knowledge about the process's functioning. In addition, a team's resources might be able to more quickly investigate a complex problem if there is some need for urgent action. Because measurement, not organizing and managing a team, is the focus of this book, this aspect of process improvement will be given only brief treatment. A number of excellent books are available for those who wish more information on team building and management (see, e.g., Scholtes, 1988).

In order to make a team function effectively, one needs to address several questions: Who should be on the team? What training is needed for team members? How will the team divide up the work to be done? Who will keep the record of team meetings? Will a facilitator be needed to assist the team? How will team members be kept informed of progress between meetings? The question of whom to include on the team may need to be revisited on an ongoing basis. Those who are initially chosen to comprise the CQI team may find that no one on the team has enough knowledge to help the team understand the entire process. The team may have to be enlarged at a later date to include those with the missing process knowledge. Another key question deals with the use of a facilitator.

Many organizations find that trained facilitators are vital to their QI initiatives. Sometimes these individuals are consultants experienced in team facilitation skills. Other times they are internal staff members who have had formal training in the facilitation of teams. In either case, however, the role of a facilitator is to provide what Deming called "the outside view." This refers to the fact that the team is frequently so involved with the process that it has difficulty asking objectively, "Are we on the right track?" A facilitator can serve as a barometer of the team's performance, can offer suggestions on how the team's meetings can progress smoothly, and discuss which QI tools should be used at which point in the quality journey.

Clarifying the Process with Flowcharts

Among the initial tasks a CQI team needs to address is clarifying the current process. A process might be affected by a number of inputs such as people, materials, equipment, method, and the environment in which the process takes place. For example, if a manager is unhappy with the quality of the secretary's typing, the process will not be improved by merely telling the secretary to improve proficiency. The manager needs to consider the process put in place for typing as well as the skills of the secretary. For example, the quality of the computer and software that the secretary uses must be evaluated. The secretary's typing also might be affected by the way in which the manager dictates a letter or by the quality of the written copy provided to the secretary. The noise level in the office and the number of other tasks required of a secretary might also influence the quality of the typing. Managers have not been traditionally trained to consider all the inputs into a process. Instead, they have tended to focus on the person and expect that the individual has total control over the output of a process.

In addition, managers may not be sensitive to the fact that when a process deteriorates, the problems are often not always in the execution of a step, but sometimes in the hand-offs between steps (see Figure 2.2). For example, if a hospital has a problem in transferring patients promptly from the emergency room (ER) to

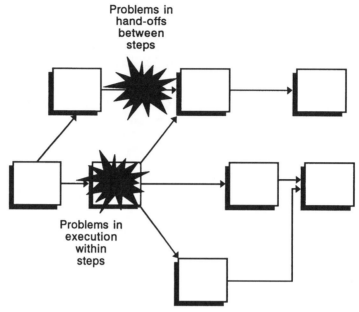

FIGURE 2.2. What can go wrong in a process?

an inpatient bed, one obvious cause of delays might be the failure of "transportation" personnel to respond quickly to requests from the ER. However, although it is true that difficulties within the transportation department itself might be part of the problem, it is equally possible that other factors outside of the control of the transportation department might have a greater impact on the process. For example, if a patient is not ready to be transported when the transportation people arrive or if the transportation department was not notified in a timely manner, these factors can have a major impact on the delay in moving a patient from the emergency department to an inpatient bed.

Therefore, if you have identified the transfer of patients from the emergency department to an inpatient bed as a process that should be improved, one of the first tasks of your team would be identifying all the steps in this process. The tool that you would use to accomplish this is the flowchart (see Figure 2.3). The first thing your team might find after making flowcharts is that the

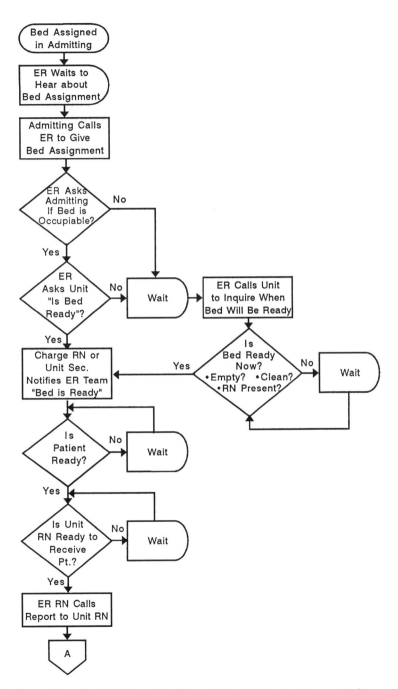

FIGURE 2.3. ER bed transfers of adults to medical/surgical units during days and afternoons only.

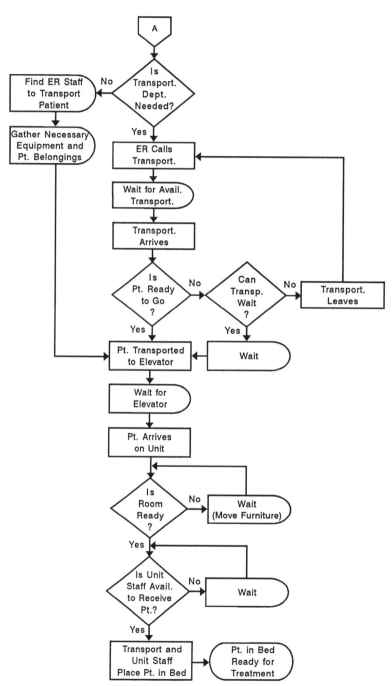

FIGURE 2.3. *(Continued)*

transfer process during the morning and afternoon shifts was different than the process used on the night shift. Therefore, your team might narrow the boundaries of the CQI project to the transfer of patients during the morning and afternoon shifts. Furthermore, because the transfer of pediatric patients is different than that of adults transferred to the medical/surgical units, you might narrow the boundaries of the process even further by addressing only the transfer of adults.

Figure 2.3 illustrates the use of various symbols in a flowchart. The boundaries of the process (i.e., the start and end of the process) are drawn in oval symbols. In the figure, "Bed assigned at admitting" is the beginning boundary and "Patient in bed and ready for treatment" is the end boundary. The various actions or steps involved in the process are drawn in rectangular boxes; for example, "Admitting calls ER to give bed assignment." Diamond symbols are reserved to identify those times in the process when a decision is to be made; for example, the "ER asks the unit if the bed is ready?" Delays in the process are symbolized by a rectangle with a curved right side. This symbol looks like a large "D," for delay.

As you study Figure 2.3, your team would discover that the transportation department was not the only, nor even the main, contributor to possible delays in transporting adults from the ER to the medical/surgical units. There were also delays in the ER itself, at the elevators, and on the inpatient units that were major contributors to the overall delay. Flowcharting a process will help you and your team to see more clearly the complexity of the process and the opportunities for improvement.

Standardizing the Process

Before you can improve a process, there has to be a uniform way in which the process is being carried out. For example, in the case just described, the team discovered that the transfer process was different for patients who came to the ER during the night shift, and that the process was not the same for adult and for pediatric patients. Therefore, the team narrowed the focus of its efforts to the transfer of adults in the morning and afternoon shifts. If the team found out that even this aspect of the transfer process was being handled in different ways, it would have to agree on performing the process in the same manner before attempting to improve it.

Identifying Key Quality Characteristics

Once your team has clarified the way in which the process currently operates, the next step is to identify the one aspect of the process you will try to improve. This aspect is referred to by some authors as the key quality characteristic (KQC). In order to identify a KQC, you first start by identifying a number of quality characteristics (QCs). These are those aspects of the process that the customer cares most about. They may vary from customer to customer, and sometimes they may conflict. For example, patients coming to an emergency room want to be treated courteously, promptly, effectively, and at a reasonable cost. They want their questions answered. If they have to be admitted, they want to be transferred to an inpatient room without delay. However, giving the best possible treatment may conflict at times with speedy service and with low cost. The team will select from among all possible quality characteristics the one it believes is the *key* quality characteristic in the view of the customer. In the example cited, the team chose "promptness" as the KQC it would address in the transfer process. It is important to realize that identifying a KQC should not be done in a vacuum by the team. They should listen to the "voice of the customer" in order to understand what the customer values. This subject is addressed in greater detail in Chapter 8.

Table 2.1 gives examples of KQCs for the processes of billing, ordering laboratory tests, and answering phones. Notice that the direct or immediate customer of each process is different, and that there are several possible KQCs that might be chosen by a CQI team.

TABLE 2.1   EXAMPLES OF KEY QUALITY CHARACTERISTICS (KQCs)

Process	Customer	KQCs
Billing	Patient	Accurate bill
		Easily understood bill
Lab tests	Physician	Timely reports
		Accurate reports
		Legible reports
Answering phones	Caller	Quick response
		Courteous treatment
		Accurate answers

Developing Operational Definitions

Having selected a KQC, the team is still not ready to collect data. KQCs are abstract concepts that need to be described in quantifiable and measurable terms. Describing a KQC in this way is called **developing an operational definition.** An operational definition gives communicable meaning to the KQC. It must be clear and unambiguous. It must specify the measurement method, equipment, and, if appropriate, the criteria by which measurement decisions will be made. It is possible to debate whether one operational definition will work better than another. But there are no "right" or "wrong" operational definitions. The key is that the operational definition must be acceptable to the team because this will guide its data collection efforts.

For example, what is a "prompt" transfer of a patient from the emergency department to an inpatient room? Fifteen minutes? Thirty minutes? One hour? Two hours? Frequently, there is no right or wrong answer to this question. However, the CQI team has to arrive at consensus on what it will consider a "prompt" admission before it can know how many patients are being admitted "promptly." Therefore, having interviewed a number of patients, the team found that the majority would become irritated if they had to wait more than 2 hours to be transferred. Therefore, the team might use the following operational definition: a "prompt" transfer is one that occurs within 2 hours or less from the time the doctor decides to admit the patient until the patient arrives on the unit and is in bed ready for treatment.

Ask yourself, for example, what operational definitions you might give to the following KQCs:

- Accuracy in delivering medications
- Courtesy in answering telephones
- Promptness in delivering food trays
- Promptness in responding to laboratory requests
- Cleanliness of a patient room

After you have developed what you think is a clear, unambiguous, and communicable definition for one or more of these KQCs, ask a colleague to do the same, and then compare your results. Chances are you will have different operational definitions. Try to resolve your differences and see whether you can arrive at a common definition that you think could be given to someone assigned to collect data.

Once you have addressed these seven issues, you should be in a good position to move on to developing a data collection plan—the topic of the next chapter.

3

Data Collection

In Chapter 2, the reader was encouraged to follow seven steps before embarking on a data collection journey. Unfortunately, many people ignore these fundamental steps and proceed from "We have a problem!" to "Let's go get some data!" All too often they forget why they are collecting data in the first place. From a CQI perspective, the goal of data collection is to gain an objective view of the process under investigation and to understand how it is performing over time.

Data versus Information

The healthcare field is replete with data. Few industries collect as much data as we do in healthcare. The problem we face, therefore, is not a data problem, it is an information problem. Austin (1983) helps to clarify the difference between these two concepts:

> [D]ata refer to raw facts and figures which are collected as parts of the normal functioning of the hospital. Information, on the other hand, is defined as data which have been processed and analyzed in a formal, intelligent way, so that the results are directly useful to those involved in the operation and management of the hospital.

In other words, data can be produced by pushing a button on a computer or by recording lab results in a patient's chart. Information, on the other hand, can be generated from data after someone asks the right questions (e.g., why has this patient's white blood count been steadily been increasing over the past 24 hours?), and places the data within its proper context. When data are placed within a framework for analysis, there is an excellent chance that information for decision making will emerge. Until this is done, however, the data will remain as facts and figures.

Figure 3.1 depicts a framework for turning data into information. This framework reflects the basic components of the scientific method (Lastrucci, 1967). It represents a process that proceeds along both inductive and deductive lines of thinking. If done in an ongoing fashion, Figure 3.1 is very similar to the Plan/Do/ Study/Act (PDSA) cycle championed by Shewhart and Deming (see Deming, 1986). By applying the scientific method to raw facts and figures, managers have a greater opportunity to make significant impacts on the processes they manage. If this type of thinking is not applied to the data we amass each day, however, it is very likely that we will be data rich, information poor, and end up wondering why we really do not understand the results of our efforts.

Components of a Data Collection Plan

Because it is done so often, it is generally assumed that data collection is a very simple thing to do. It is simple only if you ignore the various issues that need to be considered before embarking on a data collection effort. What makes collecting data even more interesting and challenging is the fact that it is as much art as it is science. You can read several books on the subject of data collection and each one will have a little different approach. The science of data collection comes from reading and studying the various tools, techniques, and methods outlined by experts in the field. The art of data collection comes from years of applying these scientific principles to real-life situations.

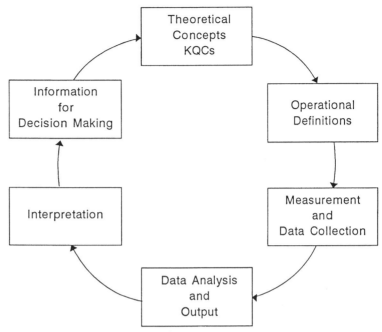

FIGURE 3.1. Framework for a data/information system.

Any good data collection effort begins with the development of a plan. This plan should address not only the technical details of how you expect to actually gather the data, but also the reasons for collecting the data and how the data will be used. The remainder of this chapter provides a series of questions and brief commentaries that should help the reader prepare a data collection plan. This list is by no means definitive. It is a practical one that we have used over the years with various research initiatives and quality improvement teams. As you review these questions, keep in mind that they should be discussed **before** you begin collecting data. Frequently, a team will dive into data collection, begin to analyze the data, and then discover that it forgot to stratify the data by shift or that its sampling approach was wrong. It seems obvious, but the time to discuss all of these questions is prior to actual collection. Again, the house painting analogy used in the last chapter is appropriate in this case. You should not expect the paint to last very long if you did not properly prepare the house before applying the paint. In the same way, you should not expect your data to produce good information for decision making if you do not dedicate yourself to thinking about the data before you collect it.

Why Do You Want to Collect These Data?

It is amazing how many strange looks you get when you ask this question. Try it the next time you are in a meeting and someone says, "Let's collect data." Just ask the person who made the proposal, "Why?" You will probably get a look that suggests that you are not in control of your faculties. Yet, if you ask this question frequently, you will find that much of the data people think they need are not essential to the decision-making process. There is a great deal of data that provide interesting facts and figures, but the real question is whether these data are essential. Asking "Why?" will get you closer to understanding what data are really essential than merely agreeing to join in a data collection frenzy.

From a quality improvement perspective, data should be collected so the team can take action. Specifically, data should be collected in order to do the following:

- Understand the variation that exists in a process
- Monitor the process over time
- See the effect of a change in the process
- Provide a common reference point
- Provide a more accurate basis for prediction

In short, data are collected in order to conduct statistical studies that provide the basis for taking action. Deming identified two types of studies that should help us understand why we are collecting data. First, he defined **enumerative** studies as those that are done on a static population for a given period of time and/or location and are designed to merely describe outcomes. Enumerative studies address the following types of questions:

- What were the average charges for this group of patients?

- What was the average length of stay and standard deviation for all hip-replacement patients last year?

- What was the percentage of surgical patients admitted last year?

The second type of study Deming identified is an **analytic** study. Analytic studies are done on dynamic processes, are not restricted to single points in time, focus on predicting the future rather than describing the past, and seek to determine why the outcomes were observed and how to improve the processes that produced the observed outcomes. In this case, the appropriate questions to ask include the following:

- What can be said about the processes that led to this group of patients having these charges?

- What can we predict about the length of stay for hip-replacement patients for the coming year?

- What were the causes of an observed decrease in surgical inpatients during the previous year?

- How will we know whether an improvement strategy will be effective?

CQI teams should be familiar with these two types of studies and when it is appropriate to conduct each type (see, e.g., Deming, 1942, 1975; Gitlow et. al., 1989). Familiarity with these concepts will be of tremendous assistance when you are asking the question, "Why do you want to collect these data?"

On What KQC Will You Be Collecting Data? How Will the KQC Be Operationally Defined?

Being very clear about the concept you are seeking to measure is crucial. Once a concept is agreed upon, you can then proceed with the development of an operational definition. The importance of selecting and specifying your KQC and its operational definition were discussed in Chapter 2.

How Often and for How Long Will You Collect Data?

This question addresses the issues of frequency (how often) and duration (how long). Will you collect data on every patient every day for the next 2 months? Or will you randomly select one patient every day and do this for 1 week in September? The choice of frequency and duration will set the stage for the quality of your data. Frequently, teams ignore these issues because they find them to be too detailed. In this case, the "Let's go get some data" orientation precludes thinking about these questions. In the long run, however, the ability of your data to adequately represent the process hinges on your responses to these two questions.

Will You Employ Sampling? If So, What Sampling Design Do You Propose?

After you answer the frequency and duration questions, the next logical step is to discuss sampling. This is not the book to provide a lengthy discourse about sampling. There are plenty of good books that accomplish this task (Selltiz et al., 1959; Blalock, 1960; Duncan, 1986; Western Electric, 1984; Gitlow et al., 1989). For our purposes, it is important to distinguish between three sampling approaches. These are depicted in Figure 3.2 and described in what follows.

Simple Random Sampling

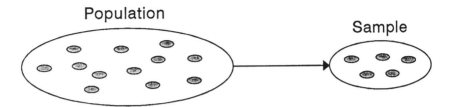

Proportional Stratified Random Sampling

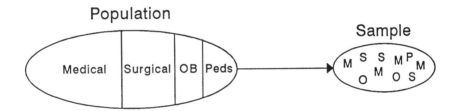

Judgment Sampling (for Analytic Studies)

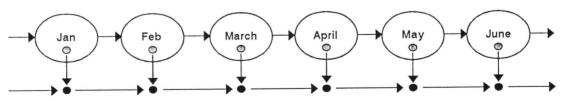

FIGURE 3.2. Sampling options.

A **simple random** approach to sampling seeks to allow every member of a population to have an equal chance of being included in the sample. In this case, a table of random numbers is usually used to facilitate the selection of the sample. This approach requires a minimum amount of knowledge about the population in advance and is free of possible classification errors.

Two major disadvantages of simple random sampling are that it (1) does not make use of knowledge of the population that the team members might have and (2) often produces larger sampling errors for the same sample size than in stratified sampling. Simple random samples are frequently drawn when the objective is to conduct an enumerative study.

The second type of sample shown in Figure 3.2 is the **proportional stratified random sample.** In this case, the total population is divided into categories or strata. In Figure 3.2, the categories represent types of patients (medical, surgical, obstetrics, and pediatrics). The proportion of cases in each category should be the same in the sample as in the population as a whole. Then a random process is used to select cases within each category.

There are clear advantages to this approach. First, it assures representation with respect to the relevant categories that form the basis of the population. Second, proportional stratified random samples produce less variability or error than a simple random sample. Third, the chances of failing to include members of each category of the population are reduced. Finally, the characteristics of each stratum can be estimated and analyzed. On the other hand, this approach has disadvantages. For example, proportional stratified random samples require accurate information on the population in each stratum. Furthermore, the costs associated with this type of sampling will usually exceed those of a simple random sample because (1) you have to make sure the strata are mutually exclusive and (2) you will need a larger overall sample to ensure an adequate number of people within each stratum.

The final approach to sampling shown in Figure 3.2 is **judgment sampling.** For Deming, this was the method of choice for conducting certain types of analytic studies, namely, those using

$\overline{X}$-R and $\overline{X}$-S charts (which are discussed in Chapter 5). Judgment sampling (also known as expert, or rational, sampling) entails selecting a series of subgroups from the population based on the opinion of those who have expert knowledge of the process. The subgroups can be drawn either by random or nonrandom procedures. In Figure 3.2, this is represented by the small black dot that is extracted from the entire population for each month. Note that the judgment sample is being drawn on a continuous basis, whereas the samples drawn by simple random and proportional stratified random procedures are for fixed points in time.

Judgment samples have the advantage of being less costly than the other approaches, require less data, and enable the team to take action on a dynamic process as it unfolds over time. On the negative side of the ledger, sampling error cannot be measured with judgment samples. Expert knowledge of the process and the population are required, and the results of a single judgment sample cannot be generalized to the population from which it was drawn. But if your objective is to take an analytic approach to process improvement, then judgment sampling should be among your sampling tools. The use of judgment samples and their place in quality studies is explained more fully by Deming (1975).

Will You Conduct a Pilot Study before Collecting Data on a Large Scale?

It is not uncommon for a team to jump into a full-scale, in-depth, data collection initiative and never even consider conducting a pilot study. Pilot studies (sometimes called pretests) provide a convenient way to identify obstacles that could have negative impacts on your data collection efforts. Think of the pilot study as a tryout to see how well your data collection plan will work. You can test your ideas and methods and determine if changes are necessary before you start full-scale implementation. For example, if you were planning on collecting data on lab turnaround time, you might want to pilot test your data collection sheet, the accuracy of the automated log-in system, and the volume of orders produced by shift and/or type of lab test. With these data, you could make adjustments to your data collection plan. Another option is to conduct the pilot study and then convene a focus group to discuss the pros and cons of the initial data collection plan. In the long run, most teams find that a pilot study is an effective way to test their ideas and plan ahead.

How Will You Collect the Data?

When you finally get to the point where you are ready to collect data, how will you do it? Will you use a data check sheet, a survey, observation, focus groups, historical records, phone interviews, or some combination of these methods? Each approach has various costs associated with it. For example, developing a data check sheet is relatively inexpensive, but the time it takes a staff person to extract the data from logs or records may be costly. Conducting focus groups requires the investment of considerable time and expense if you ask an external facilitator to conduct the sessions for you.

Because much of the data maintained by healthcare providers are stored electronically, it appears, on the surface at least, that these will be easy and inexpensive data to retrieve. Many teams have found the situation to be just the opposite, however. Healthcare data systems are usually created to (1) handle billing issues, (2) deal with administrative processes, or (3) record the history of what happens to a patient. Most healthcare databases have not been created to answer CQI questions. So teams will be faced with using either existing data systems and being satisfied with proxy measures or creating a new database that addresses their specific needs.

A related question is: Who will be responsible for gathering the data and placing them on a check sheet, extracting them from computer files, or conducting focus groups? Faced with this practical question, a team will often freeze. It realizes that it has forgotten a simple but fundamental point—someone has to do the job of assembling the data. With this realization, the team members may react by saying how busy they are. Doctors assume that the nursing staff will collect the data. Nurses think that the unit secretaries will be responsible for data collection. Unit secretaries hope that the student interns will be given this assignment, and so on. Again, the time to think about this job is before you reach this point, not as you are embarking on data collection.

A final consideration is data collection cost. How many hours of staff time will be expended? Will you have to pay for overtime? How will the data generated during the afternoon and evening shifts be collected? Sooner or later all initiatives must face the dreaded question, "How much?" An estimate of the cost of data collection will be essential for the team and its sponsors.

Will This Data Collection Effort Have Any Negative Impacts on Patients, Staff, or the Families of Patients?

Most hospitals and health systems have some form of an institutional review board (IRB) that monitors various data collection and research activities. Many CQI initiatives will not be relevant to an IRB's scrutiny, but it is important to discuss whether the data collection endeavor will have any negative impacts on those who come in contact with the process being studied.

How Will the Data Be Coded, Edited, Verified, and Analyzed?

If you think data collection is messy, then wait until you have to code, edit, verify, and analyze the data. These are the activities that most people assume will be handled by someone else: internal quality consultants, information systems staff, or summer interns sponsored by the research and education department. Perhaps, one of these groups will be able to lend assistance, but do not count on others to do the work that should be done by the team. One of the aspects of CQI that has made it work successfully for manufacturing companies has been that the team has taken responsibility for data analysis. It is reasonable to obtain internal consultation from those who are skilled in the techniques of database creation and statistical analysis, but the team must take ownership of its data and its analysis.

How Will the Data Be Used and Who Will Have Access to the Raw Data and the Results?

It is very easy to become so wrapped up in the data collection process that you do not stop and consider maintaining security for the data. Confidentiality of patient records and information is one of the most sacred trusts we have as healthcare professionals. The team must make sure that it has a consistent perspective toward confidentiality and data disclosure. Increasingly, some legal experts have even posed the question as to whether the data collected by a CQI team are fair game under the discoverability laws. This warning is not intended to make team members paranoid about data collection. It is merely intended to serve as a cautionary note. As the public, purchaser groups, and the press continue to make demands for healthcare data, we all must be aware of what we can and cannot do with the data we collect.

A Template for Data Collection

The questions just posed should guide your data collection discussions. What you need, however, is a framework, or template, for organizing the results of all these discussions into an actual plan. Table 3.1 provides such a template. You should feel free to add or revise columns in this matrix to suit your own data collection needs. Basically, you need to design a format that allows you to convey to relevant audiences the components of your data collection plan and how you intend to implement them. The example shown in Table 3.1 reflects the work of a team whose goal was to develop a measurement plan for its trauma system. You can see that it (1) identified the relevant measures or concepts it wished to measure; (2) developed an operational definition for each measure; (3) specified the data sources, individuals, and departments responsible for achieving the various tasks; and (4) provided space for additional comments. This format worked well for this team. What you need to do is decide what works best for your team and then modify this template for your own use.

TABLE 3.1   TRAUMA MEASUREMENT TEAM: DATA COLLECTION PLAN

Key Concept	Specific Measures	Operational Definitions	Data Source(s)	Collection • Schedule • Method • Responsibility	Collaborating Department/ Division/Program	Priority/Comments
Clinical outcomes	Functional outcomes following trauma sign-off	Functional outcome is defined as the patient's level of independence in daily self care, mobility, and communication as measured by the Functional Independence Measure (FIM) within 24-hour consult, trauma sign-off, rehab discharge, and 90 days post-rehab discharge.	FIM score on Uniform Data Set (UDS) reporting sheets	1. FIM rating forms completed on all trauma patients within 24 hours of rehab consult by trauma RNs. 2. Interim FIM ratings completed by appropriate RN within 24 hours of rehab admission. 3. Hospital scores completed within 24 hours of rehab discharge by designated therapists. 4. Follow-up FIM rating completed by 6W program office 90 days post. Data collection sheets to be developed. Collected on a quarterly basis.	• Rehab • Nursing	Steps 2–4 Are part of current rehab program evaluation and dictated by UDS agreement. Timing and raters may not be changed.

TABLE 3.1 (continued)

Key Concept	Specific Measures	Operational Definitions	Data Source(s)	Collection • Schedule • Method • Responsibility	Collaborating Department/ Division/Program	Priority/Comments
Resource optimization	Acute care LOS	LOS will be tracked for each person admitted as an inpatient (excluding rehab and psych patients) as recorded in the trauma registry log book. LOS will be measured in whole days counted at midnight per the registration system, including day of admission and excluding day of discharge.	Registration system and the case-mix system	• Check on a daily basis using midnight as the determining factor. • Finance Dept. and Trauma Dept. will be responsible for collecting the data.	• Admitting Office • Units • ER • Finance Dept.	Prior to developing control charts or other forms of analysis, the Trauma Measurement Team should decide on satisfaction levels to apply to the LOS measure.

4

Understanding Variation

No two people are alike! No two snowflakes are the same! Things always change! Every patient is different! These comments are common in our culture and demonstrate that we do understand variation. Or do we? We seem to acknowledge that variation exists in certain aspects of our lives, but ignore its presence in others. For example, we recognize (but may not like) the fact that variation exists in our bowling, golf, or racquetball games. We acknowledge the fact that our commutes to work are not always the same. We even concede that our children are not all alike in their abilities, talents, or interests. Yet, when it comes to thinking about variation in the workplace, we seem to have a slightly different perspective.

Many people who readily acknowledge variation in their private lives fail to acknowledge the presence of variation in the workplace. Why, for example, do some managers look at monthly budget statements and react one way when the numbers are positive and another way when there are negative variances? Why does a negative 2.3 percent change in hospital admissions from April to May send shock waves through the hospital? Why do hospital administrators get excited when the volume of procedures drops for three consecutive months? The answer to these questions is actually quite simple—people really do not understand variation! Wheeler (1993: vi) offers a potential reason for this situation:

Managers and workers, educators and students, accountants and businessmen, financial analysts and bankers, doctors and nurses, and especially lawyers and journalists all have one thing in common. They come out of their educational experience knowing how to add, subtract, multiply, and divide; yet they have no understanding of how to digest numbers to extract knowledge that may be locked up inside the data. In fact, this shortcoming is also seen, to a lesser extent, among engineers and scientists. This deficiency has been called "numerical illiteracy."

Throughout the remainder of his book, Wheeler builds an argument that the best way to overcome this deficiency and "extract knowledge" from data is to understand variation.

Depicting Variation

There are basically two options for depicting variation: (1) static displays and (2) dynamic displays. Historically, the dominant approach to depicting variation has been to use static displays. A **static display** of variation occurs when data are presented in tabular fashion, when measures of central tendency (the mean, median, and mode) and measures of dispersion (the range, standard deviation, variance, coefficient of variation, etc.) are calculated, and when data are shown in aggregated fashions (e.g., in tables, bar charts, or histograms). A **dynamic display** occurs when the data are plotted on run or control charts. A dynamic display allows you to see how the data vary over time. Static displays of data can be compared to taking a snapshot with a camera. Dynamic displays, on the other hand, are more like the moving picture obtained with a video camcorder. Each approach has its place and purpose. Your challenge is to know when to use each approach and understand the degree to which each type of display allows you to unlock the knowledge that is hiding inside the data.

The best way to demonstrate these two approaches and the knowledge that can be gleaned from each one is by example.

Imagine that you are the manager of a family practice clinic. You have been collecting patient satisfaction surveys for the past 6 months and discovered that the one item that is consistently the number one complaint is the wait time to see a physician. Your staff nurse tells you that the wait times do not seem very long. The employee who schedules appointments tells you, however, that the patients always seem bothered by the amount of time they have to wait to see a physician. So, what do you do with these two views of variation? The correct answer is, nothing! If you rely on anecdotal information (especially that which is based on only two observations), you will probably make the wrong decision.

What you should do is collect data on patient wait time. You direct your staff to collect data on patient wait time, and after 1 week, you are ready to analyze the data. If you choose a static display approach to understanding variation, you would probably produce a tabular summary similar to that shown in Table 4.1 or a graphic display shown in Figure 4.1. The numbers shown in Table 4.1 are preferable over a single statistic such as average wait time, but they still do not reveal much about the variation in the process. These numbers **describe** the process but do not depict the variation over time. If all you wanted to do was to describe the process to someone, this table would be adequate. If you want to improve it, however, this table is inadequate. If you decide to use the histogram shown in Figure 4.1, you gain more insight than merely using numeric summaries, but you are still looking at data in a static fashion.

TABLE 4.1   PATIENT WAIT TIME

Number of patients seen	150
Average wait time	45.1 minutes
Median wait time	32.6 minutes
Minimum wait time	7.3 minutes
Maximum wait time	94.5 minutes
Range	87.2 minutes
Standard deviation	16.2 minutes

No. of Patients (n = 150)

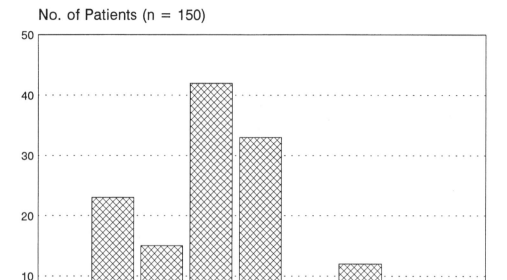

FIGURE 4.1. Patient wait time to see a physician.

Histograms are often used by managers to portray variation, so Figure 4.1 requires further commentary. How does this type of display help you make better management decisions about the variation in this process? For example, what is the longest wait time? All you know is that it is over 80 minutes. What is the shortest wait time? Again, all you know is that it is less than 10 minutes. Although this display provides some information and can lead you to ask many questions, it has severe limitations for improving patient wait time.

An alternative approach would be to display the variation in a dynamic fashion, as shown in Figure 4.2. In this case, you can see that the data are displayed over time. You observe that Mondays often have the highest average wait times, and that Wednesdays frequently have the lowest average wait times. The highest aver-

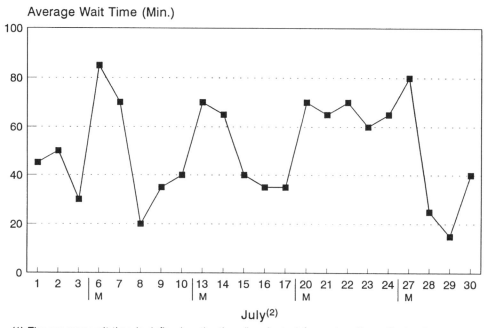

(1) The average wait time is defined as the time (in minutes) from when the patient arrives at the front desk until the patient is seen by a physician.
(2) Note that the data were collected only for weekdays.

FIGURE 4.2. Average wait time by day (July 1992).

age wait time was observed after a holiday (July 4th). Finally, you note that these data are only for weekdays and that an operational definition of "wait time" has been developed for measurement purposes.

The dynamic display has some advantages over the static display. By using dynamic displays you can (1) decide if common or special causes of variation are present and (2) ask questions to help understand the process and enhance further data collection and analysis. The question of whether common or special causes of variation exist in these data will be answered in the next chapter when run charts are discussed. In terms of asking additional questions, however, there are several that the clinic's practice manager might raise:

- What were the staffing patterns each day?

- What was the volume of patients each day? (Remember that the numbers plotted in Figure 4.2 represent "average wait time" by day. You do not know how many patients were seen each day and the average wait time could be concealing a great deal of variation within a day.)

- What type of visits were these? Were they primarily well-baby visits, school physicals, or follow-up appointments for earlier visits?

- How does patient volume vary by hour of the day?

Most management decisions are based on static displays of variation rather than on dynamic displays. Yet the processes managers are trying to understand are dynamic in nature, not static. Wheeler offers a similar perspective, "Much of the managerial data in use today consists of aggregated counts. Such data tend to be virtually useless in identifying the nature of problems" (1993: 84–85). Although a dynamic display of variation should not be used every time you wish to depict variation, it is the preferable approach if you are genuinely interested in improving process performance.

Common versus Special Causes of Variation

Walter Shewhart was the first to distinguish these two types of variation. In his original work, however, he referred to controlled or "chance" causes of variation and uncontrolled or "assignable" causes of variation. It was Deming who, in the late 1940s, coined the terms "common" and "special" causes of variation. Deming (1986: 310) writes:

Shewhart used the term assignable cause of variation where I use the term special cause. I prefer the adjective special for cause that is specific to some group of workers, or to a particular production worker, or to a specific machine, or to a specific local condition. The word to use is not important; the concept is, and this is one of the great accomplishments that Dr. Shewhart gave to the world.

Common-cause variation is an inherent part of every process. It is random and is due to regular, natural, or ordinary causes. Common-cause variation affects all outcomes of a process and results from the regular rhythm of a process. It produces processes that are stable, or "in control." One can make predictions, within limits, about a process that has only common-cause variation.

Special-cause variation, on the other hand, is due to irregular or unnatural causes that are not inherent in a process. Special-cause variation affects some, but not necessarily all, outcomes of a process. When special causes are present, a process will be "out of control," or unstable. A process also will be unpredictable if special causes are present.

The basic points that both Shewhart and Deming were trying to make were (1) variation exists in all that we do, (2) processes that exhibit common or chance causes of variation are predictable within statistical limits, (3) special causes of variation should be identified and eliminated, (4) attempting to improve processes that contain special causes will increase variation and waste resources, and (5) once special causes have been eliminated, it is appropriate to consider changing the process.

An example should help to clarify the difference between the two types of variation. Suppose that the average number of patient falls per month at your hospital for the last 2 years was 31. Sometimes an individual month may have gone as high as 39, and at other times it went as low as 25. Yet, few staff were concerned that this was anything out of the ordinary. In fact, your risk management department has historically reported this range of figures to the quality assurance (QA) committee and no one ever questioned the data or the process. Then, three months ago, the number of falls started to go up. First it was 45, then 49, and finally last month it was 53. Upon seeing these figures, the chair of the QA committee concluded that the last three data points reflect a "trend." You are at a loss in terms of explaining the increase because you do not know whether the observed variation is "noise" that is part of the "normal" variation of the patient fall process or whether the variation is truly a "signal" that the process is "out of control" as some have suggested.

So, what do you do? Do you acquiesce and agree with the QA chair because you do not want to question authority? Do you contend that the data are flawed and that you really need several more months to see if this is really a process out of control? Obviously, neither of these answers is the correct line of thinking. What you would want to do is to determine whether the process is exhibiting common or special causes of variation. Only after addressing this issue can you (should you) feel comfortable with answering the question: Is this process out of control? The challenge for management, therefore, is to know how to identify common from special causes of variation and make decisions that are appropriate for each type of variation.

Consequences of Not Understanding Variation

The first thing that happens when people do not understand variation is that they **see trends where there are no trends.** How many data points does it take to make a trend? Most people would say that it takes more than one data point to make a trend. But, what about two data points in a row that go up or down? Does this constitute a trend? How about three? Four? For sure, five data points must constitute a trend? Right? Well, the answer is, maybe. Statistically, there is an answer to this question and it will be discussed in the next chapter. For now, however, it is sufficient to realize that most managers will see a "trend" in the data long before one actually exists. You may want to see a trend, or you may honestly believe that a set of data actually reveals a trend, but in most cases, the "trend" will exist in your mind's eye, not in the data.

The second behavior that people exhibit when they do not understand variation is to **blame and give credit to others for things over which they have little or no control.** Imagine, for example, that you are in charge of the admitting department for a large hospital. You observe that last week your staff averaged 22 minutes to admit elective surgery patients (i.e., the time from when the patient arrives in the admitting area until he/she is transported onto the unit, placed in a bed, and is ready for treatment). You are very pleased with this result and to show your appreciation, you buy pizza for your staff to celebrate. The next week, however, you discover that the average admission time jumped to an average of 43 minutes for the same type of patients. How could this be? Especially after you bought pizza! You decide that action has to be taken. You call everyone to a special meeting and tell them that they must work harder and achieve the old average of 22 minutes. You tell them that if the average is not brought down, you will be forced to crack down on them. What you are unaware of is that your staff worked just as hard when the average was 43 minutes as when the average was 22 minutes. The reason that there was such a difference between the two weeks was due not to the workers, but to other things going on that affect the admission process (e.g., census variations, transportation staff attending a seminar, and construction delays on several floors). If you do not understand variation, you will inevitably blame and give credit to people for things over which they have no control.

Third, failure to understand variation will **build barriers, decrease morale, and create an atmosphere of fear.** As people make the wrong conclusions about the sources of variation, they will inevitably look for someone to blame when things do not go well (see the previous point). This sets up an environment of "we" versus "they." If workers know that the boss will use the variation in the data to reward and punish them, then their sense of loyalty and respect will be minimized. They will live in fear, wondering when they will be called into "the office" to explain why the process is not meeting expectations. Faced with these possibilities, people will either distort the system that produced the numbers or distort the actual data rather than tolerate abusive behavior.

Finally, if you do not understand variation, you will **never be able to fully understand past performance, make predictions**

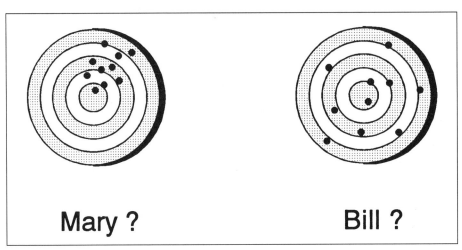

FIGURE 4.3. Who is the better shot?

about the future, and make significant improvements in your processes. Figure 4.3 sheds light on this final point. This figure shows how two individuals, Mary and Bill, placed 10 shots on a target. Which individual is the better shot? Most people would say Mary is the better shot because she has her shots clustered. Bill may have hit the bull's-eye, but his pattern is so erratic that it will be difficult for us to predict where his next shot will land, or how we can make improvements in his accuracy. Mary, on the other hand, merely has to adjust her sights down and to the left. Then, her shots should all cluster near the center of the target. All too often, people take the most current data point and assume that this represents the process's performance. If you are really sincere about understanding where your processes have been, where they are now, and where they can be in the future, you must become knowledgeable about the types of variation and how to depict them.

5

Using Run and Control Charts to Analyze Process Variation

Understanding variation from a conceptual point of view provides only a start. If a team is truly interested in quality improvement, it must take action to improve something. Run and control charts provide the basis for taking action. This chapter provides an overview of the basic principles behind using run and control charts to analyze process variation. Because run charts require no statistical calculations, can be developed quickly, and are usually not addressed in standard Statistical Process Control (SPC) texts, both the use and construction of a run chart are covered.

Control charts, on the other hand, do require statistical calculations and are documented extensively in most SPC texts (see, e.g., Duncan, 1986; Pyzdek, 1990; Montgomery, 1991; Western Electric, 1984; Wheeler and Chambers, 1992). For these reasons, we discuss only the use of, theory behind, and types of control charts in this chapter. In the Appendix, the various formulas for calculating the control limits for five frequently used control charts are presented for reference purposes. The particulars of actually constructing a control chart, however, are left to the reader.

Constructing Run Charts

A run chart provides a running record of a process over time. It offers a dynamic display of the data and can be used on virtually any type of data (e.g., counts of events, percentages, and dollars). Because run charts require no statistical calculations, such as sigma limits, they can be understood easily by everyone on the team. The major drawback in using run charts, however, is that they can detect some but not all special causes. This point will become more apparent when we discuss examples of run charts.

The following steps should be followed in order to construct a run chart:

- Draw a horizontal line (the X-axis) and label it with the unit of time (day, week, or month) or the sequence in which the data were collected.

- Draw a vertical line (the Y-axis) and scale it to cover the full range of current data plus sufficient room to accommodate future data points. A rule of thumb is to extend the Y-axis by ±20 percent of the range of the data.

- Plot a minimum of 15 data points on the graph in time order.

- Connect the points on the graph with a solid line.

- Determine the median for the data and draw it on the graph.[1] The easiest way to determine the median is to first find the **median position** by taking the total number of data points, adding 1, and dividing this number by 2. This will let you know where the median is located in the data set. For example, if there are 24 data points, the median position is (24 + 1) / 2 = 12.5.

---

[1]While some authors, such as Torki (1992), advocate using the mean for the center line of a run chart, we prefer the median because it provides a good estimate of central tendency, whether the data are normally distributed or are in a skewed distribution. Pyzdek (1990) also advises using the median for constructing run charts.

- Next, take a piece of paper, start at the top of the graph, and slide it down the plot of the data. Each time you reveal a data point, place a check mark next to it. Continue to reveal data points until you reach the median position. For the example given with 24 data points, the median position is 12.5, which means the median falls between the twelfth and thirteenth data points. Draw a line horizontal to the X-axis at the median position. The median line is typically identified as $\tilde{X}$. This is the point at which half of the data will be above the median and half of the data will be below it. As a check, you can reveal the data points by moving the paper up the graph and you should end up at the same location as you did when you revealed the data from the top down.

- Finally, the **median value** can be found by noting where the median line crosses the vertical, or Y-axis. Typically, the median position and the median value will not be the same. So, be sure you understand how to arrive at both of these values before moving on to analyzing and interpreting the run chart.

The first step in analyzing a run chart is to understand what is meant by a "run." **A run is defined as one or more consecutive data points on the same side of the median.** When you are counting runs, you should ignore points that fall directly on the median.

In Figure 5.1, the number of patient falls per month has been plotted. The median is shown as 49 and a total of 18 data points are displayed. The runs have been circled to assist the reader in analyzing this chart. The first run appears on the left side of the chart. It is a run of three data points. Because the next data point falls on the median, it is ignored. The next run also contains three data points, each of the next two runs contain two data points, and the last six runs each contain only one data point. Note that the fourth data point from the right also falls on the median.

An alternative way to count the number of runs is to count the number of times the sequence of data points crosses the median

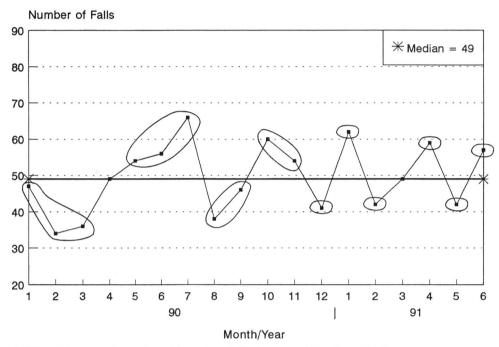

Number of Falls

FIGURE 5.1. Run chart of total inpatient falls (January 1990–June 1991).

and add 1. If you count the number of circled runs or if you add 1 to the number of times the data crosses the median, you should get the same number, 10. So, in Figure 5.1, there is a total of 10 runs.

Figure 5.2 presents data on the number of times restraints were used with a group of psychiatric patients. Whether you circle the number of runs (as shown on the graph), or count the number of times the connecting line crosses the median and then add 1, you arrive at a total of 8 runs.

Using Run Charts

The purpose of identifying the number of runs is to determine whether the process exhibits common or special causes of varia-

Number of Times Restraints Recorded

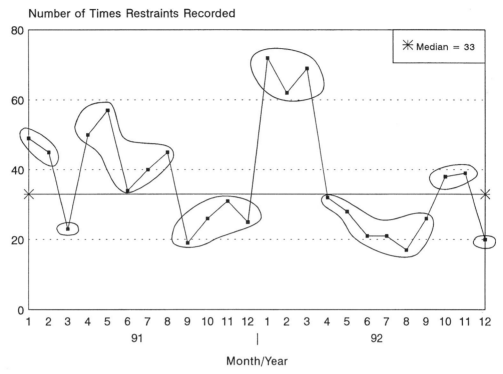

FIGURE 5.2. Run chart for the use of restraints with psychiatric patients.

tion. Four simple tests are applied to the chart to determine the source(s) of variation:

Test 1

The first test is designed to determine whether there are *too few* or *too many* runs in the data. First, calculate the number of "useful observations" by subtracting the number of data points on the median from the total number of data points. Then, find this number in Column 1 (on the next page). The lower limit for the number of runs is found in Column 2, and the upper limit is found in Column 3. If the number of runs in your data fall below the lower limit or above the upper limit, this is a signal of a special cause.

Column 1 Useful Observations	Column 2 Lower Limit	Column 3 Upper Limit
15	4	12
16	5	12
17	5	13
18	6	13
19	6	14
20	6	15
21	7	15
22	7	16
23	8	16
24	8	17
25	9	17
26	9	18
27	9	19
28	10	19
29	10	20
30	11	20
31	11	21
32	11	22
33	11	22
34	12	23
35	13	23
36	13	24
37	13	25
38	14	25
39	14	26
40	15	26

Test 2

A special cause also exists if a run contains too many data points (i.e., the run is too long). If you have less than 20 useful observations, then 7 or more data points in a run indicate a special cause. If you have 20 or more "useful observations," then 8 or more data points in a run indicates a special cause. This test identifies a shift in the process.

Test 3

A statistical trend also signals a special cause. A trend is defined as an unusually long series of consecutive increases or decreases in the data. The following table should be used to identify a trend.

Total Number of Data Points on Chart	Number of Consecutive Ascending or Descending Points Indicating a Special Cause
5 to 8	5 or more
9 to 20	6 or more
21 to 100	7 or more

For this test, you count points on the median, but ignore points that repeat the preceding value (see Pyzdek, 1990).

Test 4

Fourteen or more points in a row forming a "zig-zag" pattern constitutes a special cause. Some texts refer to this pattern as a "saw-tooth" pattern because it looks like the teeth on a saw blade.

If you go back to Figure 5.1, you can now determine whether this process reflects common or special causes of variation. You started with a total of 18 data points. Following the guidelines in Test 1, you subtract the 2 data points that fall on the median from the total and obtain 16 "useful observations." For 16 useful observations, the lower number of runs is shown to be 5 and the upper limit of runs is 12. There were 10 runs in this data, so there does not appear to be either too little or too much variation in this data.

Test 2 is designed to see whether a shift in the process has occurred. If a run is too long, it is a signal of a special cause. To apply this test, you begin with the number of useful observations again. The guideline for this test tells us that if we have fewer than 20 useful observations, we look for 7 or more data points in a run. If this occurs, then this signals a special cause. In Figure 5.1, none of the runs contains 7 or more data points. Therefore, this test is not violated and no special causes are detected.

Detecting the presence of a trend is the purpose of Test 3. Despite what many people think, 2 or even 3 points in a row do not constitute a trend. As was mentioned in the last chapter, one of the problems that occurs when people do not understand variation is that they see trends where there are no trends. Statistically, a trend is determined by the number of data points on the chart. The table presented for Test 3 shows that for 18 data points, 6 points steadily increasing or decreasing constitutes a trend. Is there such a pattern in Figure 5.1? An upward trend of 6 points is detected in the data. This signals a special cause.

Finally, Test 4 (14 points in a row switching back and forth to form a zig-zag pattern) is not detected. This test is used frequently to detect lack of stratification in data collection or the presence of tampering with the operation of a machine or a process.

If you consider all of the tests you just applied to the patient fall process, what do they tell you? The short answer is that the patient fall process, shown in Figure 5.1, is not in control. Although it exhibits a mixture of common and special causes of variation, the presence of the special cause (in this case a trend) gives us a clear signal that the process is unstable and not predictable. As will be discussed in Chapter 7, the correct action to take is to investigate the origin of the special cause and try to remove it from the process. But for now, constructing and analyzing the run chart has been sufficient. For practice, the reader is encouraged to apply the run tests to Figure 5.2. Are special causes present or is this a common cause process? The answer to this question can be found in the case study on psychiatric restraints in Chapter 6.

Using a Run Chart to Help Improve the Preadmission Testing Process

Patients admitted on the same day they are to undergo surgery (referred to as Same Day Surgery Admission—or SDSA— patients) should not have to be delayed because preadmission testing (PAT) was not done properly. Delays do not make the patient, the surgeon, or the support staff happy customers. Yet, when a team from the PAT area developed a run chart on the SDSA patients in July, they discovered that only 33 percent had completed all PAT procedures. As expected, the surgeons and support staff voiced displeasure with the process.

The results of this baseline analysis are shown on the left side of Figure 5.3. The team discovered that even though there appeared to be a considerable amount of variation in the process, it was in control. No special causes were detected, so they initiated an improvement strategy that was implemented throughout the month of August. When they collected data in September and constructed a new run chart, they found that the process had changed. Their findings are shown on the right side of Figure 5.3. These data also exhibit common-cause variation but show that the median moved from 33 to 75 percent. Although there is still further opportunity for improvement, the team was very pleased that they had been able to make things better for their customers. The run chart helped them understand (1) how the process was performing before they took action, (2) whether the process contained any special causes, and (3) the impact of their improvement strategy.

Why Use Control Charts?

Run charts are convenient, easy to understand, and can detect some special causes. But, one of their major difficulties is that they are not as sensitive in detecting special causes as control charts are. For example, the run chart will miss what are called "freak" points. These are data points that have values far above or below the majority of data points on the chart. Because the run chart's

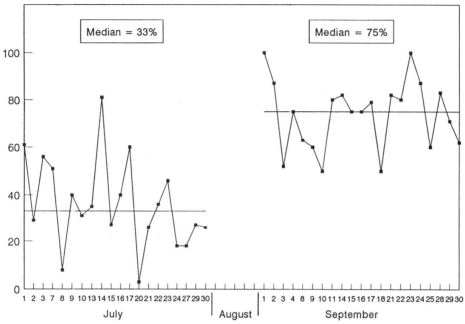

FIGURE 5.3. Preadmission testing (July–September 1992).

center line is the median, which is not sensitive to the absolute value of any single data point, freak points will be missed as special causes on a run chart. In other words, when the data have a number of extreme values, run charts will have a high probability of leading you to believe that there are no special causes when, in fact, they do exist. Another reason for using control charts is that they have the added feature of control limits, which allow you to determine the capability of the process and more accurately predict the future behavior of the process. When you use run charts, you cannot determine process capability.[2]

---

[2]We are using the expression "process capability" in a general sense to describe the amount of variation that can be expected around the center line of a control chart. Process capability is used differently in industry and in manufacturing to describe the extent to which a process meets the customer's specification limits. As we ordinarily do not have specification limits for most processes in healthcare, we do not use "process capability indices" (Cp) as is done in industry. For an extended description of process capability studies in industry, see A. V. Feigenbaum, *Total Quality Control* (1991).

The Elements of a Control Chart

The elements of a control chart are shown in Figure 5.4. Basically, a control chart looks very much like a run chart. Data are plotted in time sequence with time always presented along the horizontal, or X-, axis. The variable of interest, or key quality characteristic, is placed on the vertical, or Y-, axis. Once the data points are plotted, they are connected, just as you did for the run chart. What is different, however, is that the center line is not the median but the mean. This is typically identified as $\overline{X}$ and is referred to as "X bar." The upper control limit (UCL) and lower control limit (LCL) are the other two distinguishing characteristics of a control chart. These lines are drawn parallel to the center line. The control limits provide the basis for (1) determining the capability of the process and (2) identifying special causes.

Basic Control Chart Theory

The basic statistical principles behind the development and use of control charts were first developed by Walter A. Shewhart, during the early 1920s, while he worked at Bell Laboratories. In 1931, he

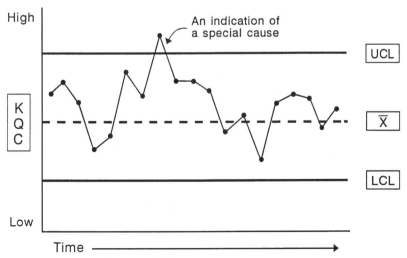

FIGURE 5.4. Elements of a control chart.

published his classic work *Economic Control of Quality of Manufactured Product*. This book has served as the foundation for all subsequent work in the field of statistical process control.

Shewhart was keenly interested in trying to understand the scientific bases for statistical control. As he observed the world around him, he realized that certain types of variation (common-cause variation) were part of the normal functioning of life. At other times, however, he observed that variation was not normal and random but due to special or assignable causes. From Shewhart's perspective, the challenge was to distinguish one type of variation from the other.

Based on this perspective, Shewhart observed:

> A phenomenon will be said to be controlled when, through the use of past experience, we can predict, at least within limits, how the phenomenon may be expected to vary in the future. Here it is understood that prediction within limits means that we can state, at least approximately, the probability that the observed phenomenon will fall within the given limits.

This definition provides a verbal description of the purpose of a control chart: prediction of the future. The question that most people ask at this point, however, is, "Okay, I understand what Shewhart is trying to tell us, but where do these control limits come from?" If you are asking this question, it is a sign that you are comfortable with the concepts and ready to proceed with some of the more technical aspects of statistical process control. If, on the other hand, you do not feel ready to explore this question, you may want to review some of the concepts presented earlier in this chapter, or those presented in Chapter 4, or you may wish to read Duncan (1986), Plsek (1992), or Wheeler and Chambers (1992).

The basis for constructing control limits is grounded in a fairly simple statistical principle. Specifically, data that exhibit common-cause variation will form a distribution that looks more or less like a bell-shaped curve. Once you know the basic shape of this distribution, you can use it as a frame of reference for future data. Plsek (1992) summarizes this point by stating:

> [C]omparing the variation in our data to the predictable pattern of a common cause system and deciding whether or not to launch a special investigation—are the essence of control chart theory.

The normal distribution is a special type of bell-shaped curve, which is shown in Figure 5.5. This curve is symmetrical and unimodal, so its mean, median, and mode will be the same value as shown by the vertical line descending from the top of the curve to the base line. The three vertical lines spaced equally on either side of the center line are referred to as standard deviations. The standard deviation is a measure of the spread or dispersion of a distribution and is usually denoted as SD, sigma, or symbolically as σ.

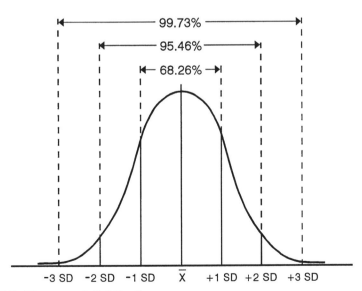

FIGURE 5.5. **The normal distribution.**

Nearly all basic statistics books describe the normal distribution in considerably more detail than is provided here. Even without a refresher course in statistics, however, most readers will remember that 68.26 percent of all data in a normal distribution will fall between ±1 SD of the mean. Similarly, 95.46 percent of the data can be found within ±2 SDs. By the time you reach ±3 SDs from the mean, you will find 99.73 percent of all the data in a normal distribution. The upper and lower control limits on a chart correspond to ±3 SDs from the mean. Statistically, this means that there is a 0.27 percent probability of having a data point fall beyond ±3 SDs of the mean (100 percent − 99.73 percent = 0.27 percent). When a data point does exceed the UCL or LCL, this is an indication of a special cause.

Figure 5.6 brings the various concepts presented in this chapter together into one diagram. It shows data plotted in time sequence and the elements of a control chart (i.e., the UCL, LCL, and the process average). It also shows how these data can form a distribution that is in the shape of a bell-shaped curve on the right side of the figure. The upper and lower control limits coincide

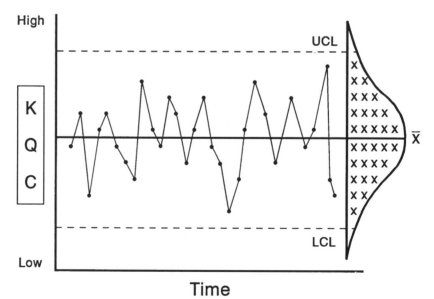

FIGURE 5.6. The relationship between a normal distribution and a control chart.

with ±3 SDs from the mean of the distribution, which is also the mean or center line for the control chart. Thus, this figure shows the relationship between the structure of the control chart and the statistical theory that serves as its foundation.

Type I and Type II Errors

The manufacturing sector has commonly used 3 sigma control limits to detect special causes. Since 2 sigma limits include approximately 95 percent of all the data under the normal curve, there is a 5 percent chance of having data fall outside ±2 sigmas. By comparison, at 3 sigmas, this percentage is reduced to 0.27 percent.

When you select limits of less than 3 sigmas, the risk of concluding that a data point requires special action when it is actually part of a common cause system, is greatly increased. This action results in committing what is called a Type I error. When people make Type I errors, they will be inclined to "tamper" with a process that is already stable.

On the other hand, a Type II error occurs when you conclude that a data point indicates no need for special action when a special cause does indeed exist. Type II errors lead to "undercontrolling" and become more frequent when the limits are made wider than ±3 sigmas. The challenge, therefore, is to balance the risk of tampering against the risk of undercontrolling. In the first case, you will see special causes when they do not exist, and, in the second case, you will miss special causes when they are present. The combined total risk of Type I and Type II errors is minimized when the 3 sigma limits are used. These relationships are depicted heuristically in Figure 5.7.

The choice of three sigma limits is not based solely on probability theory but because they work well in practice. They provide effective action limits when applied to real life situations. As Shewhart (1980: 276) says, "We must use limits such that through their use we will not waste too much time looking unnecessarily for trouble."

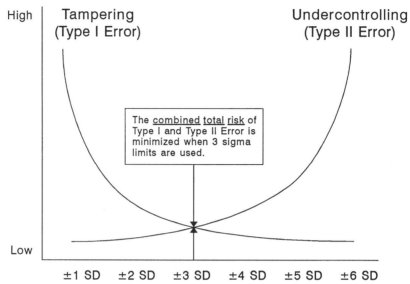

FIGURE 5.7. Balancing the risk.

In healthcare, however, it may be necessary to consider the nature of the problem when selecting sigma limits. For example, 3 sigma limits may be acceptable when dealing with late food trays or the number of days it takes to mail a patient invoice. On the other hand, physicians might feel that when patient lives are involved, they cannot wait until a data point exceeds 3 sigmas before taking action. When the well-being of patients is at risk a case can be made for using 2 sigma limits as "early warning limits." This issue has been discussed by Blumenthal (1993), but its consistent application will require further study.

Dividing a Control Chart into Zones

One of the advantages the control chart has over the run chart is that the control chart is more precise and can identify special causes that are missed in the run chart. This is accomplished by dividing the control chart into six equal zones that fall between the UCL and LCL. The zones are labeled A, B, and C, respectively, and are shown in Figure 5.8. Because the UCL and the LCL are each

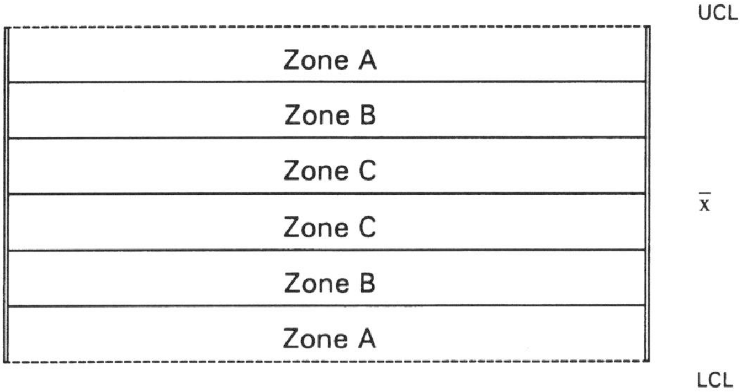

	UCL
Zone A	
Zone B	
Zone C	
Zone C	$\bar{x}$
Zone B	
Zone A	
	LCL

FIGURE 5.8. Dividing a control chart into zones. Because the center line (or mean) divides a control chart into two equal halves, it is possible to establish zones above and below the center line. Furthermore, because the control limits are 3-sigma limits, each zone is 1 sigma wide. Thus, you end up with a total of six zones. (Use of the zones to detect special causes presumes that the data plotted on the chart approximate a "normal distribution.")

3 sigmas away from the center line (for a total of 6 sigmas), each zone is equal to 1 sigma. After the zones are plotted, they can be used to identify special causes that fall between the UCL and LCL.

The tests for identifying special causes in control charts are summarized in what follows. For a more detailed explanation of these tests, see Western Electric's *Statistical Quality Control Handbook* (1984).

Apply these tests independently to **each side** of the center line:

One point outside the 3-sigma limit

Two out of three successive points in Zone A or beyond

Four out of five successive points in Zone B or beyond

Eight successive points in Zone C or beyond on the same side of the center line

Apply these tests to the **entire** chart:

Seven or more points in a row steadily increasing or decreasing indicate a trend if you have 21 or more data points (six points constitute a trend if you have less than 21 data points)

Fourteen successive points alternating up and down forming a sawtooth pattern

Fifteen consecutive points in Zone C (±1 sigma)

Although these additional tests make the control chart a more precise tool for detecting special causes, their use presumes that the data plotted on the chart approximate a normal distribution.

Deciding Which Control Chart to Use

There is basically one way to construct a run chart and that method was described earlier in this chapter. In contrast, there are numerous ways to construct control charts and calculate control limits. The challenge is to know when a particular type of chart should be used and when it should not be used. This decision hinges primarily on the type of data you have collected.

There are basically two types of data:

1. **Continuous (or variables) data** can take on different values on a continuous scale. These data either can be whole numbers or they can be expressed in terms of as many decimal places as the measuring instrument can read. Examples of continuous data include time, weight, length of stay, blood sugar levels, total number of procedures, and total number of discharges.

2. **Discrete (or attributes) data** are basically counts of events that can be aggregated into discrete categories (e.g., acceptable versus not acceptable, infected versus not infected, and late versus on time).

   It is helpful to distinguish two types of discrete data. The first type involves counting both the occurrences and the nonoccurrences and reporting the number or percentage of "defectives." An example of this is the percent of incomplete patient charts. In this case, you know the occurrences (the number of incomplete patient charts) and you know the nonoccurrences (the total number of complete patient charts). The ability to obtain both a numerator and a denominator allows you to calculate the percentage of incomplete patient charts.

There are times, however, when you know the occurrences but you do not know the nonoccurrences. This is the second type of discrete data. For example, you can count the number of patient falls during a given period of time, but you do not know how many "nonfalls" there were. Similarly, you can count the number of needle sticks, but you do not know how many "nonneedle sticks" there were. Counts of this nature are usually regarded as "defects" as compared to "defectives."

As you go about your daily activities, start asking yourself whether the data with which you come in contact with are continuous or discrete. Ask your associates if they can classify a given set of data into one of these categories and then see whether your conclusion about the data matches theirs. This is not an academic exercise. The classification decisions you make about your data will guide your selection of a particular control chart. If you conclude that your data are discrete when they are actually continuous, you will probably construct the wrong control chart. This, in turn, could lead to erroneous conclusions about common and special causes.

Once you have decided whether your data are continuous or discrete, you then have to decide which chart to construct. This is not a book about control chart construction, so the remainder of this chapter is devoted to the logic behind selecting a particular chart. The mechanics of actual chart construction can be found in any of the leading texts on SPC cited throughout this book. For reference purposes, however, we have included an Appendix with the formulas for constructing the control limits for each chart to be discussed.

Figure 5.9 presents a control chart decision tree and seven of the most frequently used control charts. Some of these chart are more appropriate to the healthcare field than others. Because

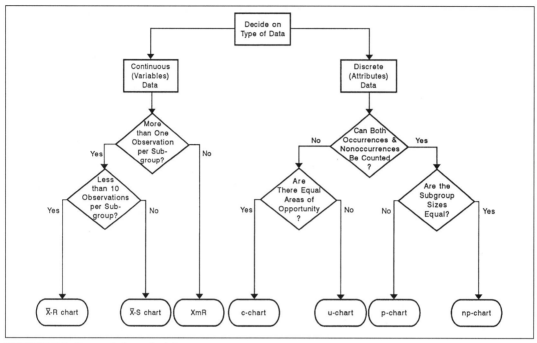

FIGURE 5.9. Control chart decision tree.

these seven are the ones most often discussed in the literature, however, the reader, at least, should be acquainted with the names of the charts and when they might be used. The case studies presented in the next chapter will provide even more insight about the application of these charts to healthcare issues.

The easiest way to follow this decision tree is to view it in two segments. First, consider the left side of the diagram. This is the side that deals with charts that are based on continuous or variables data. There are three charts that can be made with this type of data:

- The average and range chart ($\overline{X}$-R chart)

- The average and sigma chart ($\overline{X}$-S chart)

- The individual values and moving range chart (XmR chart).

The decision as to which of these charts to use depends on answering the question posed in the diamond under the block entitled "Continuous (Variables) Data" in Figure 5.9: **More than one observation per subgroup?** Before answering this question, you need to understand the nature of a subgroup. Shewhart first coined the expression by calling it a **rational subgroup.** The establishment of rational subgroups and their selection are fundamental to the construction of accurate control charts. If the subgroups are selected inappropriately, the control limits will be misleading because the variation within each subgroup is used to determine the location of the control limits on the chart.

Basically a subgroup is a sample of data pulled from the stream of data produced by a process. Because it may be impractical or very expensive to collect data on every product or service produced by the process, the rational subgroup provides a parsimonious way to represent the entire process. The general rule of thumb is that the subgroups should be selected so that if special causes exist, the chances for differences *between* subgroups will be maximized, whereas the chances for differences due to special causes *within* a subgroup will be minimized (Montgomery, 1991; Duncan, 1986). In healthcare, a rational subgroup might be based on work shift. For example, lab tests might be performed differently during the day shift than they are during the afternoon or night shift. In this case, it would not be appropriate to select a subgroup that bridged the day and afternoon shifts because the processes are different and the data would not accurately reflect either shift. Frequently, subgroups are based on time order. Shifts, hours within a shift, days, or weeks are often used to create rational subgroups because they allow you to see whether the special causes are occurring during particular periods or whether they form a cyclical pattern.

Another possibility for creating subgroups is by machine. If the lab uses six different machines to perform a particular test, for example, it would not make sense to select data from each machine and then combine the data. A better approach would be to establish subgroups of data from each machine and make separate charts for each machine. Similar applications could be devised for intravenous machines, ventilators, blood pressure cuffs, or telemetry equipment.

Now that you understand the concept of a subgroup, it is time to return to the first question in Figure 5.9 (i.e., Do you have more than one observation per subgroup?). If you collect more than one observation per subgroup, then you can make an average and range chart ($\overline{X}$-R) or an average and standard deviation chart ($\overline{X}$-S). Your decision as to which of these to construct depends on whether you collect less than or more than 10 observations per subgroup. If you collect less than 10 observations, you should make a $\overline{X}$-R chart. If you collect more than 10 observations per subgroup, an $\overline{X}$-S chart is preferable. For example, if you were studying the turnaround time (TAT) for a particular lab test and you collected four tests during each day shift (the day shift being your rational subgroup), then you would make a $\overline{X}$-R chart. If, on the other hand, you had an automated system that allowed you to collect 20 lab tests during the day shift, then you would have sufficient data to calculate a standard deviation, and the chart of choice would be the $\overline{X}$-S chart.

However, there are frequently situations where you only have one observation per subgroup. For example, you have data on the total number of radiology procedures performed each week. In this case, the week is your subgroup and the total number of procedures constitutes one observation per week. The chart that should be constructed is the individuals chart (also known as the individual values and moving range chart, or XmR chart). Another situation in which this chart would be appropriate would be for tracking an individual patient's blood pressure. If you recorded one blood pressure reading each day, your rational subgroup is a day and you have only one measure (or observation) per day. The chart of choice in this situation is the XmR chart. In the healthcare field, there are many opportunities to use this type of chart. In the next chapter, several examples of when to use this chart are provided.

Now, move over to the right side of Figure 5.9. The first block of the decision tree identifies that you have collected discrete or attributes data. When you move over to this side of the diagram, you have a choice of four different charts. Two of the charts deal with plotting *defects* (the c-chart and the u-chart). The other two charts (the p-chart and np-chart) are designed to address *defectives.*

The first decision you have to make is to determine whether you can count both the occurrences and the nonoccurrences of the event under investigation. If you say "No," then you would follow the arrow coming out of the left side of the diamond. You will notice that your ultimate choice is between making either a c-chart or a u-chart if you cannot count both the occurrences and the nonoccurrences. In this case, you will have only the occurrence of the event (e.g., the number of needle sticks, the number of patient falls, or the number of nosocomial infections) and they are usually regarded as defects. The questions that send you toward one or the other of these charts has to deal with the concept of "equal areas of opportunity."

Wheeler defines the "area of opportunity" as the background against which the count of defects must be interpreted. Before any two counts may be directly compared, they must have corresponding (i.e., equal) areas of opportunity. If the areas of opportunity are not equal, or at least approximately equal, then counts must be turned into rates before they may be meaningfully compared. This conversion from counts to rates is accomplished by dividing a count by its own area of opportunity (Wheeler and Chambers, 1992: 256). An area of opportunity might be a nursing unit. If the number of beds on the unit remained constant over the data collection period and the census for the unit also remained fairly constant, then this would be considered an equal area of opportunity for an event (e.g., a patient fall) to occur. But, if the number of beds changed and the census was fluctuating, then there would not be an equal area of opportunity for a patient fall. Under the first set of conditions, a c-chart would be made, and a u-chart would be constructed for the latter. Situations requiring the use of each of these charts are presented in the next chapter.

If both the occurrences and the nonoccurrences can be counted, then the choice is between the p-chart and the np-chart. Again, the decision for choosing one over the other will be based on whether your subgroups are of equal sizes or not. An example is the easiest way to understand this distinction. If you are interested in the C-section rate for your hospital, you will know the number of C-section deliveries (the occurrences) and the number of vaginal deliveries (the nonoccurrences). Because the number of deliveries will vary by month, you will not have equal subgroups. One month will have 157 deliveries, the next month there will be 210, and the third month will show a total of 190. When the subgroups are not equal, the appropriate chart is the p-chart. If the subgroups are equal, the np-chart should be constructed.

TABLE 5.1   THE CHOICE OF A CONTROL CHART DEPENDS ON THE PROBLEM AND HOW IT IS STRUCTURED

Type of Chart	Medication Production Analysis
$\overline{X}$-R chart	For a daily sample of 5 medication orders, what is the TAT?
$\overline{X}$-S chart	For a daily sample of 25 medication orders, what is the TAT?
XmR chart	How many medication orders do we process each week?
c-chart	For a sample of 100 medication orders each week, how many errors (defects) are observed?
u-chart	For all medication orders each week, how many errors (defects) are observed?
p-chart	For all medication orders each week, what percentage have one or more errors (i.e., are defective)?
np-chart	For a sample of 100 medication orders each week, how many have one or more errors (i.e., are defective)?

The choice of a control chart is not always a clear-cut decision. There is a fair degree of art associated with the science of SPC. Application of the decision tree to your own situations is one of the best ways to test your understanding of these principles. Frequently, the questions you ask about the data or the problem will be of great assistance in using the decision tree shown in Figure 5.9. For example, Table 5.1 shows how the same topic, medication production, could be analyzed by using each of the seven types of charts. The choice of one chart over the other will depend on the type of data collected, on the manner in which the subgroups are constructed, and on the areas of opportunity.

Although all of these decision rules might seem a little confusing, the reader should not be discouraged. It is often more difficult to understand the verbal description of chart selection than it is to actually make and analyze a chart. If this is your first exposure to control charts, you may want to read more detailed descriptions about the charts and their use. The texts by Pyzdek (1990) and Wheeler and Chambers (1992) provide excellent starting points. The next chapter should help to clarify the criteria used to select a chart and how you go about analyzing the chart once it has been constructed.

6

Control Chart Case Studies

"I was never very good at statistics!" This statement is heard frequently when the topic of control charts is discussed. It is unfortunate, but many people apparently have had negative experiences with statistics courses in the past. These less-than-positive encounters seem to have led not only to a dislike for statistics as a discipline, but also to a lack of interest in applying statistical thinking to the world in which we live. This chapter has been developed to apply the principles of quality improvement to situations that occur every day within the healthcare field. It is more concerned with **statistical thinking,** therefore, than with formulas and mathematics.

Applying Statistical Thinking to Healthcare Processes

Each day, healthcare professionals make numerous decisions about clinical, administrative, and operational processes. But, how do they know the decisions they are making are correct? Do the processes under study exhibit common or special causes of variation? Are the processes "in control" or "out of control?" What will happen if managers conclude that their processes reflect common causes of variation when they actually have a combination of both common and special causes of variation? Answers to these questions do not come merely from making a run or control chart, but from understanding how the data were collected and how to make sense out of all the numbers. The art of statistical thinking, therefore, requires that healthcare professionals:

- Listen to the voice of the customer

- Make sure they really understand what the customer is trying to tell them

- Develop clear, objective, and measurable operational definitions

- Collect the appropriate type and amount of data

- Select a chart (run or control) that is appropriate for the type of data collected

- Interpret the results correctly

- Make a management decision that aligns the process with the voice of the customer

Case Studies

The twelve case studies presented in this chapter have been designed to demonstrate how data can be successfully transformed into information for decision making. This transformation results not so much from wrestling with the intricacies of statistical formulas, but rather from applying quality improvement principles to healthcare problems. The following case studies address clinical, operational, and financial aspects of healthcare delivery. They have been developed to assist the reader in analyzing and interpreting control charts. Although some technical aspects of control chart construction are covered, these case studies do not require any computations or actual chart construction. The challenge is to apply statistical thinking, process knowledge, experience, and good old common sense to the problem presented. Each case study is divided into four sections, as follows:

- *The Situation:* A brief scenario is presented that explains why the customers are concerned with the current process. If applicable, past history, stories, and/or data are discussed. The objective of this section is to develop a context for the case study.

- *The Questions:* A series of questions are presented with every case study. These questions will guide the reader through the chart, the data, and the decision-making challenges. The reader is encouraged to answer each question prior to moving on to the next section. Note that the questions are numbered. These numbers provide a cross-reference to the answers found in the *Analysis and Interpretation* section.

- *Analysis and Interpretation:* In this section, answers to the questions in the previous section will be provided. Some of the answers will be technical in nature (e.g., when to re-compute the upper and lower control limits), and others will be content-oriented (e.g., the reasons why a special cause exists).

- *Management Considerations:* The final section for each case study discusses some of the potential issues that managers need to consider before taking action on the process. Questions such as "When should I intervene in the process?" or "Should I collect more data?" are discussed.

CASE STUDY 1: ANALYZING THE NET OPERATING MARGIN

The Situation

You are a member of the board of trustees at two hospitals (Hospital A and B). You have information that leads you to suspect that Hospital A is well-managed and in solid financial condition, whereas Hospital B has shown indications of being poorly managed and in unstable financial condition. In September 1993, you received the first-quarter financial report for FY94 from Hospital A (shown in Table 6.1). You are puzzled because the net operating

TABLE 6.1   FINANCIAL REPORT TO THE BOARD OF TRUSTEES (HOSPITAL A)

Consolidated Key Financial Indicators
for 1st Quarter FY94

	FY 92 (7/91–6/92)	FY 93 (7/92–6/93)	1st Quarter FY 94 (7/93–9/93)	Current Goal	Long-Term Goal	S&P Median for Hospitals Rated A
Operations:						
Operating margin	3.8%	4.3%	5.6%	5.3%	7.8%	5.9%
Net return on assets	3.4%	4.1%	4.3%	3.5%	5.8%	6.5%
Liquidity:						
Days of cash on hand	103.2	105.9	141.4	>110	>160	>90
Debt coverage:						
Debt service coverage	2.54	2.80	2.72	>2.84	>4.50	>2.57
Debt to capitalization	69.1%	74.3%	76.03%	<66.0%	<41.0%	<45.0%

TABLE 6.2   NET OPERATING MARGIN (%)*
FROM JANUARY 1992 TO SEPTEMBER 1993 (HOSPITAL A)

01/92	02/92	03/92	04/92	05/92	06/92	07/92	08/92	09/92	10/92	11/92	12/92
3.43	2.88	5.33	3.62	4.59	9.27	2.80	2.44	4.79	4.97	6.22	9.04

01/93	02/93	03/93	04/93	05/93	06/93	07/93	08/93	09/93
5.49	4.45	10.15	3.03	0.27	-2.87	4.38	5.94	6.48

*Net operating margin = (Operating income—expenses) / Operating income

margins (NOMs) for FY92, FY93, and the first quarter of FY94 are *identical* to the NOMs from Hospital B, which you suspect is financially unstable.

In an effort to resolve your puzzlement, you ask both Hospital A and B to provide you with a control chart displaying their NOM by month beginning with January 1992. Hospital A sends you the actual monthly figures (Table 6.2), as well as the control chart shown in Figure 6.1. Hospital B sends you the control chart shown in Figure 6.2.

The Questions

1. What kind of data are financial ratios? Variables or attributes?

2. Why is an XmR chart appropriate for displaying financial ratios?

3. Based on Table 6.1, what can you say regarding the financial condition of Hospital A. What can you predict regarding the NOM for the remainder of FY94?

4. What is the probability of either hospital making its long-term NOM goal of 7.8 percent?

5. To what extent did the monthly NOM figures provided in Table 6.2 help you predict the NOM for FY94. What additional information did the control chart (Figure 6.1) provide you that Table 6.2 did not?

6. Without knowledge of statistical process control theory, what mistake might the management of Hospital A have made in June 1993 after seeing the NOM drop for three consecutive months, and even show a loss for the first time in June 1993?

7. Were you correct in your suspicion that the two hospitals were not in the same financial condition even though the average NOM figures were identical?

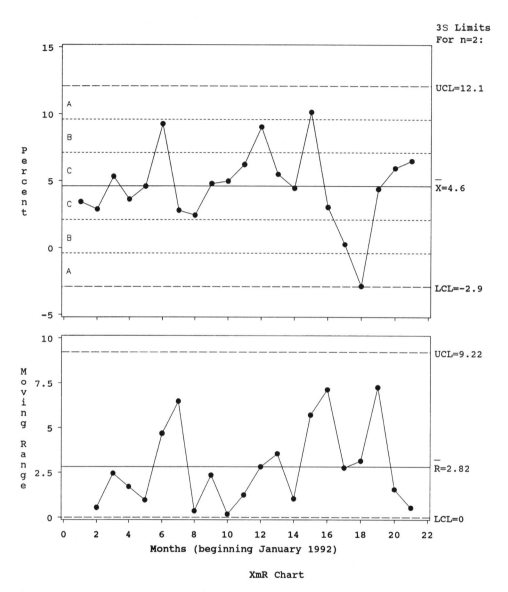

FIGURE 6.1. Net operating margin for Hospital A (for 21 months from January 1992 to September 1993).

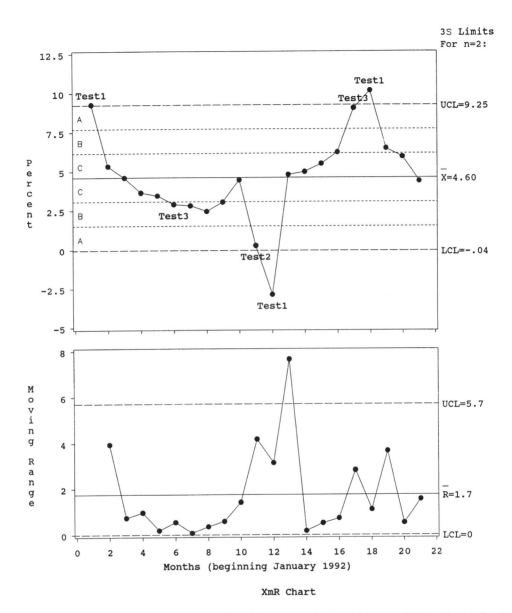

FIGURE 6.2. Net operating margin for Hospital B (for 21 months from January 1992 to September 1993).

Analysis and Interpretation

1. Financial ratios are properly considered to be variables data because they can be measured on a continuum with as many decimal places as are appropriate.

2. The XmR chart is appropriate to display monthly financial ratios because each "subgroup" consists of an individual value for each month.

3. Based on Table 6.1, your best guess is that Hospital A is in reasonably stable financial order. The NOM improved from FY92 to FY93, and the first quarter of FY94 seems to show continued improvement. However, you do not have data regarding the first quarter of the previous two fiscal years, therefore, it is possible that the first quarter of the other years were equally strong. The long-term NOM goal of 7.8 percent seems to be rather high, but you cannot be certain that it is completely out of reach. Standard and Poor's median for A rated hospitals is 5.9 percent, which is above the three reported NOM figures. However, it is not clear whether this is a valid benchmark or whether the current level of operations can reach this level during the coming months.

4. The definition of "long-term" goal has not been clearly defined. Is this goal for the coming year? For 5 years from now? For 10 years from now? Is there any plan in place that will bring the current level of operations from the 5.6 percent reported for the current quarter to the long-term goal of 7.8 percent? Based on the information provided, you cannot make any assessment regarding your hospital's ability to reach the long-term goal. It would seem on the surface to be an **arbitrary** numerical goal. As Deming would ask, "By what method do you expect to reach this goal?"

5. The NOM figures provided in Table 6.2 by Hospital A showed you that there was considerable variability from

month to month. It also revealed that there was a period of sharp decline in the NOM from March 1993 (10.15 percent) to June 1993 (a 2.87 percent net operating loss). It also showed that there was a turnaround in the first quarter of FY94, and that this quarter was considerably higher than the first quarter of the previous year. However, Table 6.2 does not help you to predict what your NOM will be for the coming fiscal year. On the other hand, the control chart provided with Table 6.1 shows that you can expect to average 4.6 percent NOM during the coming fiscal year, and in any individual month, Hospital A might show as much as 12 percent NOM, or a *loss* of 2.9 percent.

6. Without knowledge of statistical process control theory, the management of Hospital A might have experienced panic in June 1993 after seeing their NOM drop from 10.15 percent in March to a loss of 2.87 percent in June. At this point, the management might well have decided to eliminate management or staff positions, cut various services, cancel planned travel, or cut back on capital expenditures. However, managers who understand control chart theory would not overreact to a downward pattern in the data.

7. Indeed, your suspicion that the two hospitals were not in the same condition, even though the average NOM figures were identical, was absolutely correct. Figure 6.2 shows that the NOM for Hospital B is completely unpredictable. There were many indications of special causes: a drop in profit for 7 consecutive months (Test 3), eight or more points in a row below the average (Test 2), as well as several points beyond the 3-sigma limits (Test 1). The monthly figures for NOM are so unstable that one cannot predict what to expect for the rest of FY94. The control charts showed that while the average NOM for 21 months was 4.6 percent for both Hospitals A and B, Hospital B was not in stable condition. This instability would not have been

noticed if the data had been displayed in a format similar to Table 6.1.

Management Considerations

It is not always possible to make solid management decisions by merely looking at tabular data showing paired comparisons without seeing the context from which the numbers were taken. The use of tables showing summary statistics (such as Table 6.1) is appropriate only *after* one is certain that the given process is in control. In this example, Hospital A can legitimately use a tabular presentation such as that in Table 6.1, whereas Hospital B cannot legitimately do so because its process is not in control.

Finally, the use of *arbitrary* numerical goals should be avoided. Hospital A will not achieve a NOM of 7.8 percent (its long-term goal) unless some plan is put into place to change the current level of operations. Once a plan is implemented, a control chart can be used to determine the extent to which the plan is successful. To use numerical goals to "motivate" hospital management to improve will only have the negative effect of causing managers to feel defeated.

CASE STUDY 2: CBC LABORATORY TURNAROUND TIME

The Situation

Ever since you moved your lab to a new location in the hospital, several ER physicians have been complaining about the turnaround time (TAT) for complete blood counts (CBCs). They feel that the TATs have been constantly increasing for these tests and several contend that the process for obtaining lab test results is "out of control!"

You have not heard these complaints from all the ER physicians, so you decide to see whether the perceptions of those who are not satisfied with the process are valid. You decide to do this by developing a control chart on the CBC turnaround-time process.

The first thing you do is discuss the issue with your staff. You decide that the best thing to do is to understand the variation in the current process and see whether the concerns of the ER physicians are justified. The development of a data collection plan is your next step. You decide that a judgment sample of three CBCs each day should be sufficient. The data were collected for 23 consecutive weekdays. (You decide to exclude weekend data because the lab follows a different process on weekends.)

Turnaround time for a CBC is defined as the number of minutes elapsed from the time the ER physician writes the order until the result is entered into the computer in the lab. The ER ties directly into the same computer, so there is no need to send a hard copy of the results back to the ER. The test is "completed," therefore, when the result is entered into the lab computer terminal. Figure 6.3 presents the $\overline{X}$-R chart developed by one of your staff members.

The Questions

1. The control chart selected for these data was the $\overline{X}$-R chart. Was this decision correct? If you think this is the correct chart, what factors led you to this conclusion? Could another type of chart have been constructed?

2. Is the process "out of control" as some of the ER physicians have maintained?

3. What is the capability of the current process?

4. Why is there an average and a range chart? Why do you need both of these? Do they tell you the same thing?

5. So, what do you do with these charts? How will this information help you make the ER physicians more satisfied with the TATs?

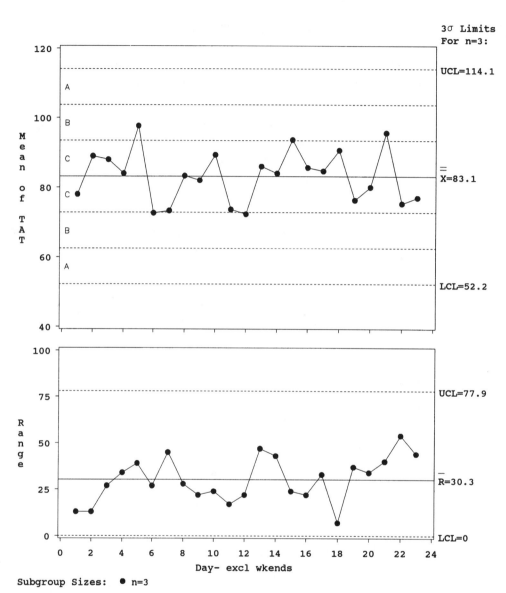

FIGURE 6.3. CBC turnaround time.

Analysis and Interpretation

1. Because the variable of interest is minutes, these data should be viewed as continuous. As can be seen from the control chart decision tree (found in Chapter 5), the correct choice is the $\overline{X}$-R chart because the subgroup size (i.e., the number of CBC tests analyzed each day) is less than 10. If the subgroup size had been 10 or more CBC tests, then the appropriate chart would have been the $\overline{X}$-S chart.

2. Even though several of the ER physicians seem to believe that the CBC TAT process is "out of control," the control chart shows that the process is in statistical control and exhibits only common-cause variation.

3. The capability of the current process is defined by the process average and the control limits. The process exhibits only common-cause variation, so we can conclude that this process will continue to take, on the average, approximately 83 minutes to process a CBC. Furthermore, the process may take as much as 114.1 minutes or as little as 52.2 minutes and still be in control (i.e., this variation reflects only normal or random variation in the process).

4. For the $\overline{X}$-R, $\overline{X}$-S, and the XmR charts, two charts are always generated. The average chart (the chart on the top of the page) reveals how the process varies between samples. The range chart (found at the bottom of the page) shows the amount of variability within the samples. When analyzing these charts, the range charts should be analyzed first. If the range chart has one or more points exceeding a control limit, you should not analyze the individuals chart (the top chart). This is because the average of the ranges is used to compute the limits for the individuals chart. If the range chart is out of control, then the UCL and LCL of the average chart will be biased. Also notice that the range chart does not have zones, because zones are not appropriate for

the range chart. Finally, note that the patterns of both charts are different. This is because they do tell you different things and should be analyzed separately.[1]

5. Several years ago, a nationally known hamburger chain employed an elderly white-haired woman named Clara to ask the question, "Where's the beef?" The equivalent question in terms of quality improvement is, "So, what do I do with this chart now that it is constructed?" Actually, answering this question is the most difficult part of the quality improvement journey. In the case of the CBC turn-around time, you know several things: (1) the process is in control; (2) on the average, it will take about 83 minutes to process a CBC in the future if nothing is done to change the current process or if special causes do not occur; and (3) the ER physicians will continue to be dissatisfied unless you use these data to show them how the process will perform in the future. If they decide that the current process average is not acceptable, then you have one basic option: Take action to improve the process!

Management Considerations

Although this analysis has been able to show how the current process is actually functioning, it raises as many questions as it answers. For example, the data reflect the total amount of time to process a CBC. Does this time differ by shift, day of the week, staffing patterns, or machine used to process the lab order? Fre-

---

[1]The use, application, and interpretation of the range chart can raise some confusion. This topic is discussed in detail by Wheeler and Chambers (1992). Readers interested in the subtleties of this issue should refer to this reference. Another technical concern is whether to use the median range or the average range to calculate the limits of the XmR chart. Most statisticians suggest using the average range unless the range chart is out of control (i.e., one or more points above the UCL) or two-thirds or more of the range values are below the average range. In either case, use the median range to compute the control limits for the XmR chart.

quently, stratifying the data can help to shed light on aspects of a process that seem to be quite confounded.

Another option might be to divide the total turnaround time into its component steps. For example, it might be useful to divide the total time into (1) the time from when the physician writes the order until it arrives in the lab (the up-front time), and (2) the time the lab takes to perform the test, enter the result into the computer, and send it back to the ER (processing time). Charts could be made for the up-front time and the process time. This might reveal that one step takes longer than another or that one of the steps is in control and stable whereas the other is out of control. Aggregate data oftentimes can mask special causes. When you divide the process into its constituent parts, you can gain new insights and make significant progress toward process improvement.

CASE STUDY 3: TRACKING THE SUCCESS OF PHYSICAL THERAPY

The Situation

You are the director of a hospital physical therapy department. The medical director of the inpatient physical rehabilitation unit has asked to meet with you periodically to review the utilization of selected procedures and therapies. In several weeks, you will be meeting to discuss the "appropriate" amount of therapy for patients who have total hip- or knee-replacement surgery. The major question for discussion will be: How much therapy is needed for these patients? The medical director is interested in keeping therapy to a minimum without jeopardizing the health or functional status of the patient. So, how much is enough?

Over the past 6 months, your staff has been asking this same question. In fact, two of the physical therapists have been curious about this issue and devised a way to measure the progress of individual patients. They believe that their approach could be of assistance in answering these questions. The basic idea is to measure the time it takes a patient to walk a fixed distance. Before therapy begins, the time it takes a patient to walk the fixed distance will be recorded and plotted on a chart. Then as the patient undergoes therapy, the patient's progress can be checked against the initial measures. The therapists actually got the basic idea for this study from Deming (1986: 252–253). The therapists took Deming's example and designed the following procedure:

- A fixed distance was laid out on the floor of the physical therapy department.

- The time for the left foot to move from floor to floor at each step was recorded by electronic impulse.

- Five successive steps (the eleventh through fifteenth steps in 20 steps) provided an average time for each patient.

- Twelve such series of observations on one patient were recorded over a period of days.

- Then the therapists worked to enhance the patient's ability to walk, and 12 more observations of five steps were recorded.

Figures 6.4 and 6.5 show the data for one patient before and after therapy.

The Questions

1. The KQC in this study is speed in walking. Are walking times considered variables or attributes data?

2. The therapists constructed an $\overline{X}$-R chart. Why did they select this type of chart? What other chart option(s) could they have pursued?

3. What additional information does the range chart tell you?

4. Are there any special causes present in either chart?

5. Can the improvement observed in the second set of charts (Figure 6.5) be attributed exclusively to the physical therapy treatments?

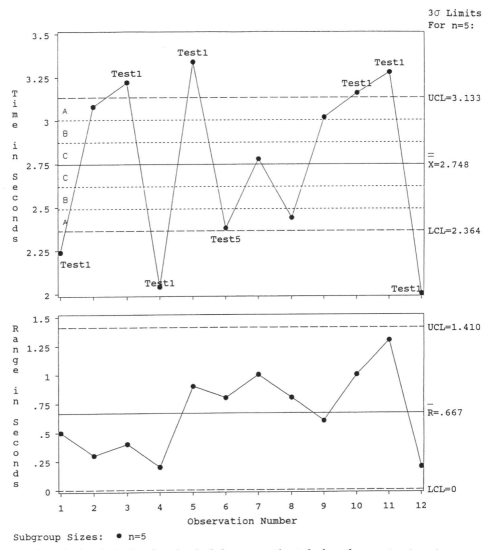

FIGURE 6.4. **Speed of ambulation for physical therapy patients before therapy treatments.**

6. What can you predict about this patient's speed of ambulation if no further therapy is provided?

7. Can you decide from these data whether further therapy is indicated? How would you use this data to answer the questions raised by the medical director?

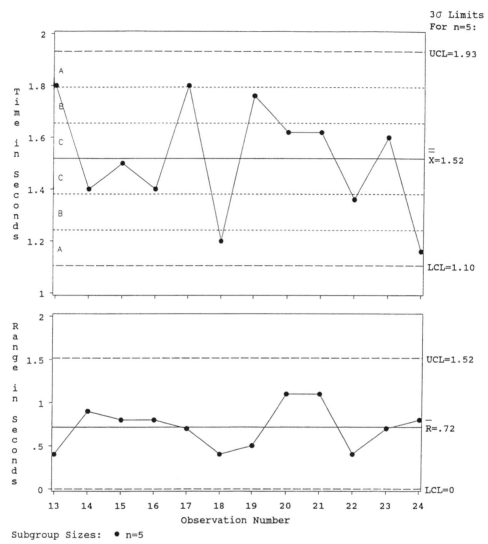

FIGURE 6.5. Speed of ambulation for physical therapy patients after therapy treatments.

Analysis and Interpretation

1. Because ambulation is measured in units of time, it is always regarded as variables data.

2. An $\overline{X}$-R chart was constructed because (1) variables data were collected, (2) there were subgroups of data with more

than one observation per subgroup (i.e., during each data collection period, five steps were recorded), and (3) the subgroups contained less than 10 observations. If the time had been recorded for 10 or more steps for each subgroup, an $\overline{X}$-S chart would be a better option.

3. The range chart (bottom chart) reveals the amount of variability within each set of five observations. The average chart shows the amount of variability between subgroup averages.

4. The data shown in Figure 6.4 (before therapy) reveal several special causes, whereas there are no special causes present in Figure 6.5 (after therapy).

5. It is clear that something happened between the first and second charts. The second chart not only is in control, but it also exhibits a process average that is much lower than the average in the first chart. Whether this difference is due *exclusively* to the physical therapy treatments, however, is debatable. For example, the patient may have been on pain management drugs during the initial testing, which could have influenced the patterns shown in Figure 6.4. It is also possible that the patient was not mentally prepared to be tested and found the whole experience to be so disruptive that it affected performance. These issues should be discussed by those who have process knowledge about this topic and understand the particulars of this patient's case.

6. If this patient does not receive any more therapy, you can predict that he will average about 1.5 seconds between steps. On any given day, the average might range from 1.1 seconds (the LCL) to 1.9 seconds (the UCL). Although you cannot predict the speed of the next set of observations, you can predict that the variability of this patient's gait by using the upper and lower control limits.

7. Is further therapy needed? This is the key question. It is also the question that the medical director will be waiting for you

to answer. The answer lies not so much with the control chart, but rather with the knowledge and experience of the therapists. The charts provide data on the capability of this patient. As Deming says in his example, "The therapist provides lessons to the patient so long as lessons help him, but halts lessons when continuation would not help him. In other words, the control chart protects the patient and makes the best use of the time of the therapist." In this case, the medical director can see that this patient's gait is predictable. Is this the best that this patient can be? If the patient is a 40-year-old male who is a marathon runner, maybe he can improve further. But if the patient is a 70-year-old male with comorbid conditions, this may be his best level of performance. Again, knowledge of the patient and knowledge of what the charts are telling you will give the kind of information needed to work effectively with the medical director.

Management Considerations

As the level of managed care continues to grow in this country, providers will be asked to demonstrate how treatments and services are contributing to increasing the quality of care while maintaining or reducing costs. This example shows how control charts can be applied to individual patient care. The key learning point is that the charts must be applied with a liberal dose of common sense and subject knowledge. Without understanding the particulars of this case, it would be difficult to say whether the patient needed (or wanted) further therapy. The fact that the chart showed that the patient's gait was stable does not mean that further therapy would not be of value.

CASE STUDY 4: DAYS TO MAIL A PATIENT INVOICE

The Situation

As director of patient billing services you have heard several complaints from your staff about the amount of time required to complete and mail a patient invoice. Some of them have even been heard to complain that the process is "totally out of control!" In order to analyze this process, you decide to collect some data. You do not control the process by which the U.S. Postal Service delivers the invoices, so you decided to address only that portion of the process you do control, namely, the time it takes to complete and mail a patient invoice. Data are collected on the number of days it took to complete and mail the last 25 consecutive patient invoices. These data were then placed on the control charts shown in Figure 6.6.

The Questions

1. The control charts selected for these data were the charts for individual values and moving ranges (the XmR chart). Are these charts appropriate for this type of data? If not, what type of chart would you recommend using?

2. Is the process "totally out of control" as some have contended? Is the patient invoice process predictable?

3. What is the capability of this process?

4. In Figure 6.6, is there a difference between points A and B? Point A (35 days) is certainly higher than point B (24 days). Should you call everybody to a meeting on the day when point A was recorded and tell them they better not let this happen again? Would it be appropriate for management to buy pizza and celebrate on the day when the low point was recorded? Does the sharp decrease indicate that there has been a change in the process?

5. How would you determine whether a planned change in the process will be effective?

6. How do you use the moving range chart (the lower chart in Figure 6.6) to understand the process? Why do you even need the range chart?

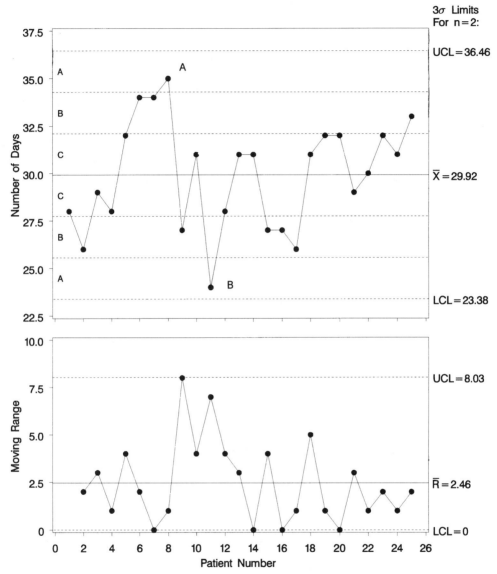

FIGURE 6.6. Days to mail a patient invoice (XmR chart).

Analysis and Interpretation

1. The KQC in this process is the timeliness of mailing a patient invoice. For the purposes of this case study, "timeliness" has been operationally defined as *the number of work days it took to complete and mail a patient invoice after the patient's service, procedure, or exam had been finished and the chart had been signed and sent to the billing department for processing.* Because days should be regarded as variables or continuous data rather than attributes data, the choice of the appropriate chart is limited to three types of charts:

   - average and range chart ($\overline{X}$-R)

   - average and sigma chart ($\overline{X}$-S)

   - individuals and moving range chart (XmR)

   As can be seen from the control chart decision tree (found in Chapter 5), the correct choice is the XmR chart because there is only one observation per subgroup.

2. Contrary to popular belief, the process is not "totally out of control!" In fact, the process is actually in control and exhibits only common-cause variation. All of the data points fall between the UCL and LCL. Furthermore, none of the zone tests for detection of special causes has been violated. Therefore, this is a predictable process.

3. What the voice of the process has told us is that, on the average, it takes about 30 days to complete and mail a patient invoice. The process capability can vary from a low of 23.38 days to a high of 36.46, and this reflects normal or common causes of variation in the process. We can predict, therefore, that the process will continue to operate within these limits until (1) something happens that signals a special cause or (2) action is taken to intervene and process improvement is initiated.

4. In terms of understanding process performance, there is no difference between points A and B. In absolute terms, they are different. But in terms of understanding variation in a process, there is absolutely no difference between them. Both are random points that are part of a common-cause process. Therefore, if you reacted in a negative manner to point A and a positive way to point B, you would be making the wrong decision.

5. If you decide to take action to improve this common-cause process, you will know you have been successful in improving the process if (1) the variability in the process is reduced (i.e., the distance between the UCL and the LCL is reduced) and/or (2) the process average moves below 29.92. In order to test the impact of your intervention, you would "freeze" the control limits and process average where they are and continue to plot new data against these values. You should not recalculate the limits every time you add a new data point. If your intervention strategy works, you will see a reduction in the variability and/or a shift in the process.

6. Finally, the moving range chart (the lower chart in Figure 6.6) is actually the first chart you should analyze. Notice that this chart does not have zones. This is because zones are not appropriate for the moving range chart. To use this chart correctly, first focus on the UCL. If a data point exceeds the UCL, you should not analyze the individuals chart (the top chart in Figure 6.6). This is because the average of the moving ranges is used to compute the limits for the individuals chart. Thus, if the range chart is out of control, then the limits of the individuals chart will be biased.

Management Considerations

Probably the most significant point in this case study is the way managers deal with points A and B. All to often, we are quick to pass judgment on a data point we do not like. When people react to a single data point (either favorably or unfavorably), they are failing to understand variation and its impact on the process. This failure inevitably leads to tampering, which will increase variation.

Another important consideration in this case study is the amount of data used in this analysis. The case study includes 25 data points. What time period do these invoices cover? Should the invoices be stratified by payer class, procedure, or diagnosis? Maybe all invoices are not alike? Do not become so enamored with the construction of the charts that you lose sight of the important interaction that occurs among your data collection plan, your data displays, and the conclusions you derive.

CASE 5: ADMISSION TIME INTO AN INTENSIVE CARE UNIT[2]

The Situation

You are the manager of your hospital's intensive care unit (ICU). For several months, you have had growing concerns about the length of time it takes to receive open heart surgery patients into the ICU. You have observed that it often takes over 30 minutes for the staff to switch over all the tubes and monitors for patients entering the ICU. To more accurately understand the switchover process, you decided to plot the switchover time for 16 consecutive patients during the month of January (Figure 6.7). Then you called a meeting of the ICU staff and showed them this control chart, which showed an average admission time of 26 minutes with a UCL of almost 44 minutes and a LCL of nearly 9 minutes. Your staff decided that this average time was putting patients at risk and that something had to be done.

Initial discussions with your staff revealed that the morning and afternoon shifts were not following the same admission

---

[2]This case study is an adaptation of a real CQI project conducted by the ICU staff at Parkview Episcopal Hospital in Pueblo, Colorado.

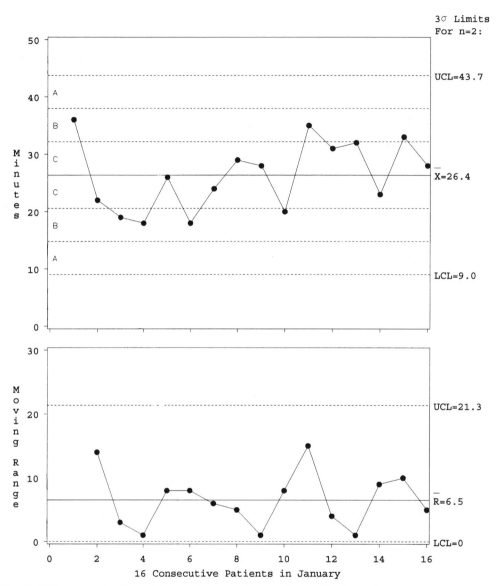

FIGURE 6.7. ICU admission time for open heart surgery patients (XmR chart).

process. The team agreed to standardize the process by developing a common protocol before making any major changes in the admission process. Then data were collected on 16 additional patients during February, and the data were compared to the January patients (Figure 6.8). An improvement was observed.

Next, your staff discovered that most of the switchover time was spent handling the intravenous (IV) lines. An anesthesiologist was then invited to meet with the ICU staff. She pointed out that the operating room and ICU were using different types of IV lines. The team agreed to begin using the IV lines used in the operating room, and the anesthesiologist agreed to train the ICU staff in how to handle the IV lines efficiently. This training took place during the month of March. New data were collected in April and compared to data from February (Figure 6.9). The capability of the April process after the intervention in March is displayed in Figure 6.10.

The Questions

1. What kind of data are these?

2. Why was an XmR chart used with these data?

3. What was the initial capability of the admissions process described in Figure 6.7? Was the process in control? What would you predict regarding the admission time if no changes were made in the process?

4. Describe the effect of standardizing the process as shown in Figure 6.8? Was it proper for the team to change the process after standardizing it? Why or why not?

5. Discuss the effect of the agreed-upon intervention as displayed in Figure 6.9? Was it successful? How do you know?

6. What was the capability of the admissions process after the intervention as shown in Figure 6.10? Should the team continue to try to improve the switchover time?

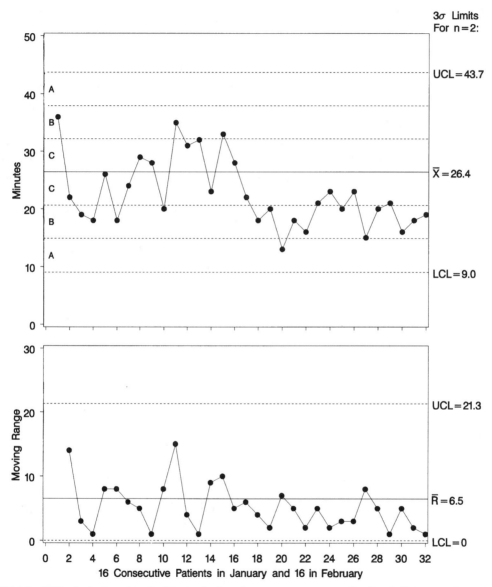

FIGURE 6.8. ICU admission time before and after the process was standardized. (Mean and control limits are based on 16 January patients.)

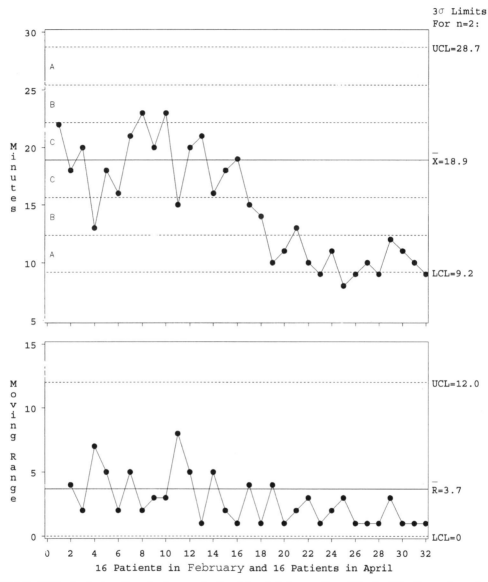

FIGURE 6.9. ICU admission time before and after March intervention. (Control limits are based on February patients.)

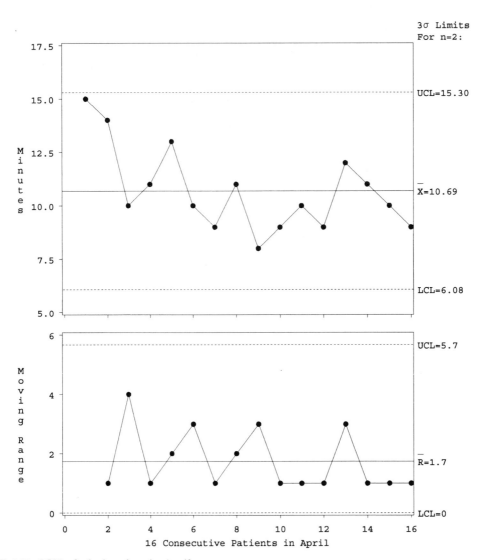

FIGURE 6.10. ICU admission time in April.

Analysis and Interpretation

1. Because the KQC is the switchover time, which is measured on a continuous scale, these data can be classified as variables data.

2. An XmR chart was used rather than an X-R chart because each subgroup is comprised of a single patient.

3. Figure 6.7 shows that the initial process was in control, that is, neither the average nor moving range charts showed any special cause. However, the process left a great deal to be desired from the standpoint of patient care, insofar as the average time for the switchover process was 26 minutes and it might take as long as 43 minutes. These numbers, along with the LCL of 9 minutes, also describe the process capability. If no changes were made in the process, these are the switchover times that could be predicted for the future. Note, that it is not possible to predict the exact switchover time for the next patient. It is possible to predict, however, the overall performance of the process.

4. Figure 6.8 shows that while the range chart is in control, standardizing the process created a special cause on the average (top) chart, that is, eight or more consecutive points below the mean showed a "shift" in the process. Perhaps the observed improvement was partially because the staff was aware that the ICU manager was recording and charting the switchover time. The capability of the process after standardization was an average of 18.9 minutes with an UCL of 28 minutes and a LCL of 9 minutes, as shown in the average (top) chart in Figure 6.9.

5. The average (top) chart in Figure 6.9 also shows that the agreed-upon intervention was successful. By using control limits for the February patients, the data for April patients clearly show a special cause. Not only were the admission

times for eight or more consecutive patients below the February mean, but the time for patients 23, 25, 26, 28, and 32 were below the LCL. The shift in the admissions process after the intervention was clearly dramatic.

6. The capability of the ICU admission process after the intervention is displayed in the average chart in Figure 6.10. The data from 16 patients collected in the month of April show that the improved process is in control with a mean of 10.6 minutes, a UCL of 15.3 minutes, and a LCL of 6 minutes. These data describe the current process. If no further changes are made, this is what can be expected for switchover times for ICU patients during the coming months. Only the quality improvement team can decide whether or not it should continue to improve the process or switch its attention to another opportunity for improvement.

Management Considerations

One of the learning points from this case study is that membership on the quality improvement team must be periodically reevaluated. Note that the quality improvement team, as it was originally constituted, had only ICU staff membership. However, to improve the process, it was necessary to invite someone outside of the ICU staff, namely, the anesthesiologist. If the team wished to continue to work on the admission process, it might have to once again add to the team membership, for example, by inviting a pharmacist to join the team.

Also note that the mean and control limits should be "frozen" whenever your team wishes to evaluate the effects of an intervention on a process that exhibits only common-cause variation. For example, Figure 6.8 illustrates how the mean and control limits for January were used to study the effect of the first intervention, that is, standardizing the process, which took place in February. Figure 6.9 illustrates the freezing of the February control limits to measure the effect of the March intervention.

If you want to know the current capability of your process, then develop control limits based on the most recent 16 to 25 data points. If the process is in control, the mean and the control limits will enable you to predict what to expect if no changes are made in the process. Once again, remember that "in control" means the process is stable and predictable. However, "in control" is not synonymous with "acceptable" or "good."

CASE STUDY 6: EMERGENCY ROOM BED TRANSFER TIME

The Situation

"Why does it take so long to get a patient from the emergency room (ER) into a bed on the inpatient unit"? Initially, only the staff in the ER asked this question. Lately, however, you have heard this question from nurses on the units, transportation staff, and patients. As administrative director of the ER, you decided that this question must be addressed. Too many of your customers have been providing negative feedback on this process. Recently, you even came across a situation where a transporter and a nurse were engaged in a shouting match over this issue.

The first thing you did was to organize an interdisciplinary team to work on this process. Some of the team members came to the meetings with preconceived notions about who was to blame for the process not working properly. With patience and assistance from a trained facilitator, you worked through some tense moments. You felt that a major breakthrough occurred when the group developed a flowchart on the current process. The flowchart enabled everyone to see that no one knew all the steps in the process and, more importantly, no individual could be singled out as the reason for the process not working efficiently.

The next step was to develop a data collection plan. The KQC (promptness) would be measured in minutes. The team decided that they could work together to collect the following time intervals:

- The time from when the ER calls admitting to say it needs an inpatient bed to when admitting assigns a bed on the unit.

- The time from when a bed is assigned by admitting until the time when the patient is in the bed on the unit and ready for treatment.

- The total time it takes to move a patient from the ER into a bed on the appropriate unit and ready for treatment, that is, the sum of the two time segments mentioned above.

Data for 31 consecutive patients were collected. A control chart was created for each of the three blocks of time and they are shown in Figures 6.11 through 6.13.

The Questions

1. The KQC in this study (promptness) would be measured by the time it takes to move a patient from the ER into a bed on the unit. Minutes are variables data (i.e., minutes can be measured on a continuous scale). In this case, whole minutes are recorded and plotted on the charts. Given that the team collected variables data, what were its options for control charts? Which type of chart was used and why was it selected?

2. What conclusions can you make from these charts? Do they all tell you the same story? If not, how do they differ? What parts of the process are in control and what parts are not?

3. What steps should the team take next?

4. Whose "fault" is it that this process does not work correctly?

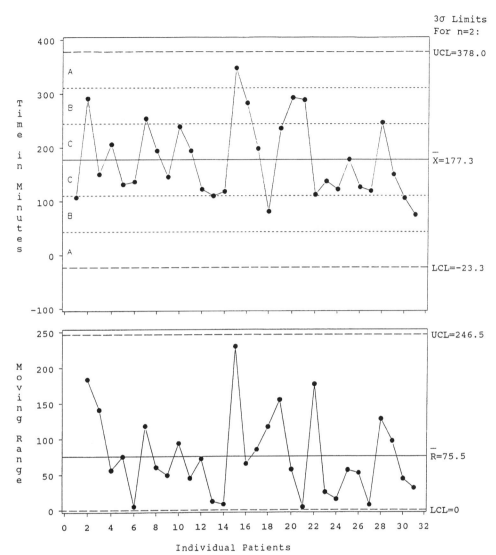

FIGURE 6.11. Total time from ER to in bed on the unit (data from August 23–27, 1993, morning and afternoon shifts).

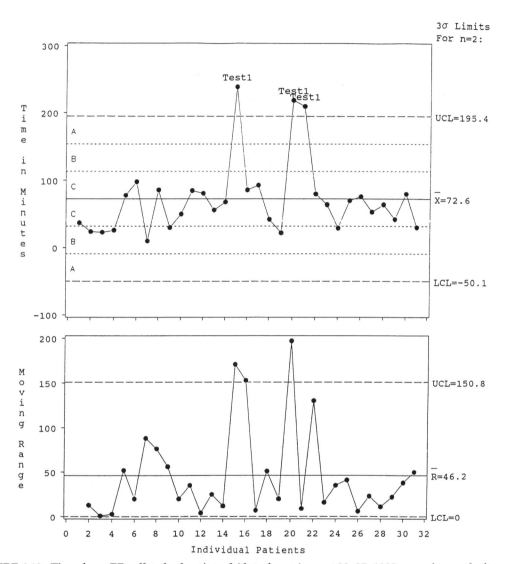

FIGURE 6.12. Time from ER call to bed assigned (data from August 23–27, 1993, morning and afternoon shifts).

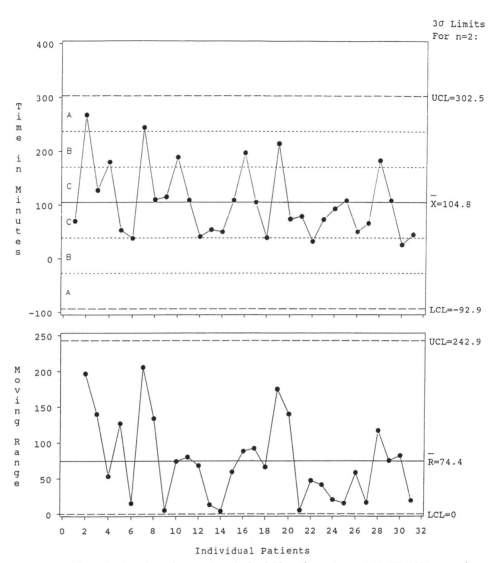

FIGURE 6.13. Time from bed assigned to patient in bed (data from August 23–27, 1993, morning and afternoon shifts).

Analysis and Interpretation

1. With variables type data, the team had the choice of making an X̄-R, X̄-S, or an XmR chart. Because they collected data on 31 consecutive patients, however, the appropriate chart is the XmR chart because each patient constitutes a subgroup of one. The other two types of charts are appropriate when there is more than one observation per subgroup.

2. The three charts do tell different stories. The first chart (Figure 6.11) shows that the bed transfer process, from start to finish, is in control. It exhibits common-cause variation and, on the average, it will take approximately 177 minutes to move a patient from the ER into a bed on the unit. The UCL is set at 378 minutes (over 6 hours). The theoretical LCL as shown is a negative number, which is not possible in this situation, so the LCL, in reality, is zero.

   Figures 6.12 and 6.13 show how the total amount of time can be divided into two major blocks. The first block is the "up-front" time (i.e., the time it takes to have a bed assigned to the patient), and the second block is the "back-end" time (i.e., the time to move the patient from the ER into a bed on the unit and ready for treatment). Figure 6.12 shows that the up-front time process is not in control. Several special causes can be seen. In this case, these special causes are related to patients whose wait times for a bed to be assigned exceeded the UCL of 195 minutes.

   The back-end time is portrayed in Figure 6.13. This step in the process is in control and has a process average of 104.8 minutes. Note that this step takes more time than the bed assignment step, which averaged about 73 minutes. When the average up-front time (72.6 minutes) is added to the average back-end time (104.8 minutes), the result is the average for the total time shown in the first chart (177.4 minutes).

3. The team decided to investigate the special causes shown in Figure 6.12 before addressing the common-cause variation

in the other two charts. During their investigation, they discovered that the admitting office was short of staff on the days when the time exceeded the UCL because five people were attending computer training. With this knowledge, the team could legitimately remove these three data points and recalculate the chart. When this is done, the data will most likely exhibit common-cause variation. Eliminating these three data points also will have an influence on the chart displaying overall time (Figure 6.11). The averages and the control limits for Figures 6.11 and 6.12 will be reduced slightly. Once the special causes are addressed, the team can decide whether it is satisfied with the amount of common-cause variation. If it is, then it would do nothing except continue to monitor the process and look for additional special causes. If, on the other hand, it does not like the variation in the current process or it is not satisfied with the process averages, then the team would need to develop an improvement strategy, implement it, and collect more data.

4. It is hoped that the team will realize that one individual cannot be singled out as being responsible for a process that does not work. It is very easy to point fingers, and in times of significant unrest, which we have in the healthcare industry today, finger pointing seems to be an easy-and-quick answer to tough questions. Clearly, the greater challenge is to help people understand how we are all responsible for our processes. Systems thinking provides the theoretical basis for enhanced responsibility and personal accountability provides the practical basis.

Management Considerations

The total time chart is in control, the second chart is not in control, and the third chart is also in control. How can the total time chart be in control when one of its parts is not in control? The answer lies in that an aggregation of data, as shown in Figure 6.11, frequently masks the variability of its component parts. When the parts are investigated on their own, however, the variability that was suppressed in the aggregate is frequently revealed. Therefore, care should be taken not to rely too heavily on the total or aggregate process times to describe how a process is functioning.

Another consideration is the application of stratification criteria to this problem. For example, should the 31 patients be placed on the same chart? Maybe it would have been revealing to stratify the patients by type of problem (car accident, gun shot, or sports injury), mode of transportation (ambulance, helicopter, or walk-in), or age. Were all of these patients admitted to the ER on a weekday or were weekends included? Does the number of tests or procedures have an affect on the amount of time required to move a patient into a bed on the unit? All of these considerations could have an impact on the way the process behaves.

CASE STUDY 7: PLATELET COUNTS

The Situation

A patient, who is to undergo an autologous bone marrow transplant for cancer, sits alone in her room reading her diary. She tries to make sense out of all the data she has recorded on her platelet counts. The platelet levels not only have been below normal, but also have exhibited rather erratic patterns of behavior. Both the patient and her physician are becoming increasingly frustrated with these patterns. Each day, numerous blood draws are taken from the patient to determine her platelet counts. Normal platelet counts should be between 200,000 and 300,000 per cubic millimeter. The last count for this patient was only 12,000.

During one of their daily meetings, the patient and her physician realize that looking at the result of each individual blood draw is not telling them very much. They decide that the individual measurements are not very helpful in determining if she is actually making progress, remaining stable, or declining. What they need is a view of the big picture. The physician suggests that it might be helpful to plot her data on a control chart. In this way, they could see how her platelet counts are responding to the various transfusions and treatments over time. The chart they developed is shown in Figure 6.14.

The Questions

1. What type of data are platelet counts?

2. The physician was not sure which type of chart he should construct. So, he consulted with the resident CQI statistician. Which type of chart do you think the statistician recommended?

3. Are there any special causes present in the chart? Is the patient's platelet process in control?

4. What could be done to enhance these charts and make them more useful to the physician's decision-making process?

5. Do you think applying control charts to individual patients is appropriate? What other clinical applications can you suggest for control charts?

Analysis and Interpretation

1. Like time, platelets can be measured along a continuous scale. This means that they should be classified as variables data.

2. The chart of choice for this data is the XmR chart. The reasons for this choice are (1) platelets are considered to be variables data and (2) each blood draw is a single or individual measure (i.e., we have a "subgroup" of one observation).

3. Figure 6.14 contains 65 data points. Three special causes are identified. Test 1 shows that one data point exceeded the UCL. Test 2 indicates that there are eight or more points in

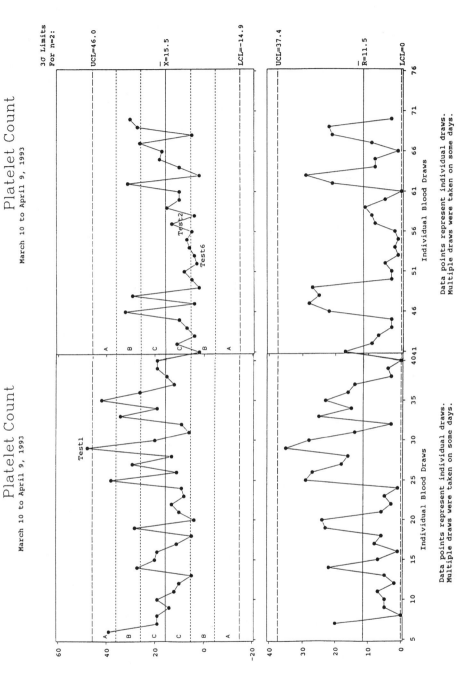

FIGURE 6.14. Platelet count (March 10 to April 9, 1993).

a row in Zone C or beyond on one side of the center line. Finally, Test 6 reveals that four out of five points are in a row in Zone B or beyond. The first special cause is clearly desirable because it shows that the patient's platelet count was at a high of nearly 48,000. This was the highest level during the entire 31-day period. This is a special cause that you would like to emulate. Unfortunately, this special cause did not last. The other two special causes relate to periods when the counts were very low. The overall conclusion is that the patient's platelet process is not stable or predictable. The goal should be to investigate the special causes, determine why they occurred, and strive to eliminate them. Once the patient's platelet count is predictable and demonstrating common-cause variation, then the physician can address how to (1) reduce the variability in her process and/or (2) move the process average in the desired direction.

4. The charts could be enhanced by annotation. Specifically, reference lines could be drawn to show each of the 31 days. In this way, the physician could see how many draws were taken each day. Notes could also be added to indicate when transfusions occurred, the type of cells administered, and when other types of drug therapies were administered. By annotating the charts, the patient and her physician could study the impacts of various treatment regimens and gain greater understanding of the interaction of the various initiatives.

5. When control charts have been applied in healthcare settings, they have typically been used to analyze administrative and managerial processes. Unfortunately, their application to the clinical practice of medicine occurs much less often. This is somewhat ironic because healthcare providers are taught that the human body consists of various systems and processes that interact and change over time. (See also

Case Study 3 describing the progress of an individual patient receiving physical therapy.) The use of control charts to analyze individual patients, therefore, is very appropriate, albeit not common practice. Control charts could be used, for example, to track the following medical conditions: hypertension, blood sugar levels, cholesterol levels, and blood clotting time.

Management Considerations

Many of the measures we take on individual patients qualify as variables or continuous types of data. This type of data allows us to construct $\overline{X}$-R, $\overline{X}$-S, or XmR charts, depending on the type of sampling that was done. As physicians and other practitioners become more familiar with the theory and tools of SPC, we should see greater application of control charts to clinical practice. In the long run, the use of control charts should enhance our understanding of individual patient processes. We should be able to see the process capability a patient has for a particular measure and be less prone to tamper with medication doses, treatments, or therapies. (See Blumenthal, 1993, for a further discussion of using control charts for tracking individual patient processes.)

CASE STUDY 8: PRIMARY CESARIAN SECTIONS

The Situation

In last evening's newspaper, an article had the following headline: "Local Hospital Reduces Primary C-Section Rate to 12%." Unfortunately, this article is not about your hospital! The hospital referenced in the article had been working for over a year to reduce its primary C-section rate (i.e., the rate of Cesarian sections done on pregnant women who have never had a C-section), which averaged about 18 percent over the past 5 years. Now that this information has been released, however, local business groups and managed care companies are asking other area hospitals to share their primary C-section rates with the public.

Historically, your hospital has developed quarterly summary statistics on your C-section rates, but none of your C-section data has ever been shared with outside groups. Your aggregated data have been displayed as histograms and compared against a "threshold" of acceptable performance that your quality assurance (QA) department obtains from obstetrics journals.

As chair of your QA committee, you need to develop a plan of action to deal with these external requests. The first thing you decide to do is to move away from the quarterly reporting of aggregated data. In its place, you recommend that the data be displayed by month and in a control chart format. You argue that this approach will not only display the data in a dynamic fashion, but also help the QA committee understand the variation in this process. The next thing you do is to agree on an operational definition of a primary C-section rate. This is defined as the total number of first-time C-sections divided by the total number of deliveries each month.

The first chart developed for the QA committee created considerable discussion. Several committee members were not happy to see the data displayed this way. They felt that the monthly primary C-section rates between August 1991 and January 1992 were higher than those for the period February to July 1991. They maintain that this represents a "shift" in the process and they are concerned that external groups will criticize the hospital for this shift. The number of deliveries and the number of primary C-sections by month for 1990, 1991, and the first quarter of 1992 are shown in Table 6.3. The chart developed from these data are presented in Figure 6.15.

The Questions

1. How would you classify C-section data? Are they variables or attributes data?

2. Which type of chart should be constructed for C-section data?

TABLE 6.3   C-SECTION DATA
(JANUARY 1990–MARCH 1992)

Month	Number of Primary C-Sections	Total Deliveries
January **1990**	65	370
February	64	383
March	77	446
April	59	454
May	64	463
June	74	431
July	72	443
August	67	451
September	59	433
October	65	407
November	60	381
December	68	406
January **1991**	62	374
February	48	355
March	57	393
April	64	417
May	66	434
June	55	421
July	51	417
August	82	444
September	65	429
October	69	411
November	62	386
December	66	357
January **1992**	58	373
February	47	370
March	59	415

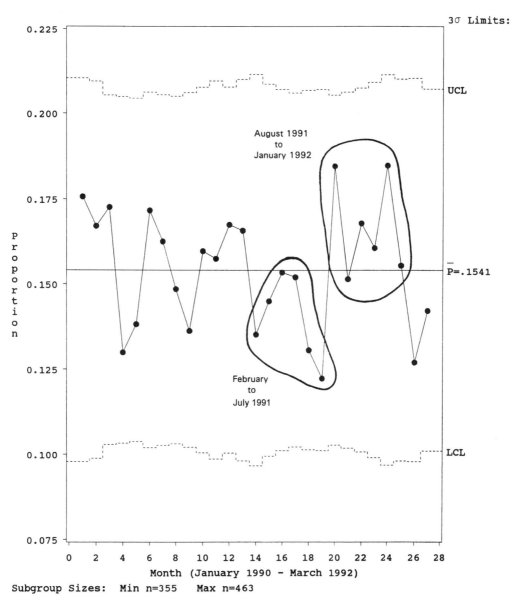

FIGURE 6.15. Proportion of primary C-sections (January 1990 to March 1992).

3. Do you agree with those on the QA committee who maintain that there has been a shift in the process?

4. What would you predict the C-section rate to be in the future if no changes are made in current obstetrics practices?

5. Why do the control limits in Figure 6.15 look like stair step? The control limits on the other charts have all been straight lines. Is there a problem with the computer software?

Analysis and Interpretation

1. The C-section data should be considered attributes data. You know the occurrences of the event (the total number of primary C-sections) and you know the nonoccurrences (the total number of vaginal deliveries). With these two numbers, you can calculate the percentage of primary C-sections during a given period of time. This is a classic example of a binomial distribution where there are only two possible outcomes: Either you have a primary C-section or you do not.

2. The appropriate type of chart is the p-chart. We know from the control chart decision tree (in Chapter 5) that there are four types of charts that are appropriate for attributes data. Because we know both the occurrences and the nonoccurrences, we have reduced our choices to the p-chart and the np-chart. The p-chart is selected because the subgroup sizes are not equal (i.e., the denominator, which is the total number of deliveries per month, varies each month). If the number of deliveries each month did not vary (which typically is not the case), then the np-chart could be created.

3. The concerns of some QA committee members are not justified. Figure 6.15 shows that the C-section process is in control and exhibits only common-cause variation. The period of concern, February to July 1991 compared to August 1991 through January 1992, does not reflect a "shift in the process." Some data points are below the process average be-

cause other data points are above the average. This is typical of random variation. Those who see shifts in the data when they do not exist are demonstrating a lack of statistical thinking. They may want to see a shift, but a careful analysis of the chart will actually tell you whether such a shift exists.

4. If nothing is done to change this process, you can expect to see about 15 percent primary C-sections each month. Because the process is in control, we know that the process will continue to operate like this until (1) special causes occur or (2) action is taken to reduce the variability in the process or move the process average in a more desirable direction.

5. The irregular, stair-step appearance of the control limits is typical of a p-chart. This is because the denominators (number of deliveries per month) vary for each data point. When the denominators are small, the control limits will be wider. As the denominators become larger, the limits will become tighter. You can test this principle by comparing the denominators for each month with the width of the limits for each month. Calculation of stair-step control limits is a real challenge by hand. For example, in this present case study, there are 27 data points. This means that you would have to compute 27 individual control limits. The best way to deal with p-charts, therefore, is with a computer. If you do not have SPC software, you can use the average of the denominators to compute straight control limits. If you choose to use the average of the denominators, however, you should become familiar with the potential difficulties that this approach has for interpreting the charts. For further reading on this issue, consult Pyzdek (1990: 121–130) and Western Electric Company (1984: 17–21).

Management Considerations

There are many variables in healthcare that are appropriate for p-charts. We frequently have unequal subgroup sizes and the outcomes of many of our processes can be viewed as binomial distributions. For example, test results can be accepted or rejected, a patient has an infection or does not have an infection, or a protocol was followed or not followed. In each of these cases, however, the total number of events (the denominators) varies, which makes the p-chart appropriate.

Another consideration related to p-charts is realizing that for many outcomes, it is probably not desirable to reduce the percentage of the occurrence to zero. In the case of primary C-sections, for example, is it desirable to have zero percent primary C-sections? Obstetricians would agree that is it not. Currently, however, there is a strong desire by many physicians to see C-sections kept to a minimum. But, this raises the question: What is their operational definition of "minimum?" Clearly, if the C-section rate is reduced too far, there could be an increase in neonatal or maternal deaths or complications. As the C-section rate decreases, it would be reasonable to plot the neonatal death rate or to construct a scatter diagram to show the relationship between the C-section rate and the neonatal death rate.

In summary, this example highlights the importance of considering the interaction of variables. It is not enough to merely plot a single variable and ignore the potential interaction of this variable with related variables. Furthermore, there will be occasions when it is not medically advisable to reduce a measure too far. This is where experience, knowledge, and common sense have to be blended with the statistical aspects of chart construction.

CASE STUDY 9: RANKING HOSPITALS ON PATIENT SATISFACTION

The Situation

A business group composed of major employers in your metropolitan area decided to develop a "report card" on which they would rank the seven area hospitals on quality. Patient satisfaction was chosen as one of several indicators of quality. To assess patient satisfaction, the business group hired a professional firm to survey area residents who had been admitted to these hospitals during the previous year. One question on the survey asked respondents to rate the "overall quality of care." They were asked to select one of the following five responses: excellent, very good, good, fair, or poor. The business group took the results of the survey and ranked the hospitals from highest to lowest based on the percentage of individuals responding "excellent" to the overall quality-of-care question. The results were then published in the local newspaper.

As a member of the management team at your hospital, you are quite concerned about the public's reaction to publishing this report card. To make matters worse, your hospital received the lowest rating of all seven hospitals (51 percent responding "excellent"). Subsequently, the marketing director at your hospital called the chairman of the local business group to get additional information on the study. She found out that the survey had been conducted by phone and that the number of respondents for each hospital varied from a low of 351 for your hospital to as many as 1,426 for another hospital.

Because a tabular presentation of the results inadequately portrayed the variation among the seven hospitals included in this study, the marketing director took the information she gathered on the study and developed a p-chart to display the results in a graphic fashion (see Figure 6.16). The p-chart shows that the average percent "excellent" was 56 percent, and that one hospital (hospital 7) scored above the UCL with a rating of 64 percent "excellent."

The Questions

1. Should the percentage of "excellent" ratings be considered attributes or variables data?

2. Why did the marketing director use a p-chart rather than a u-chart to display the data?

3. Why are the UCL and the LCL so uneven?

4. Why are there no lines connecting the ratings from the seven hospitals?

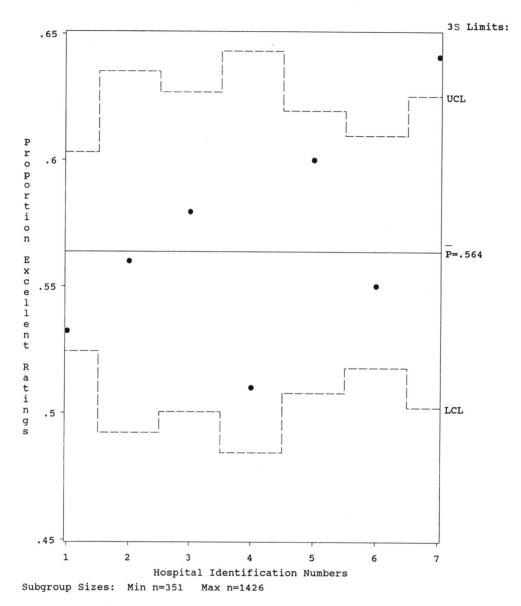

FIGURE 6.16. Proportion of excellent ratings of overall quality (survey of patients at seven hospitals conducted by a business group).

5. What questions need to be answered before you can legitimately use a p-chart to examine these data?

6. In the event that the data from the seven hospitals are reasonably comparable, how would you interpret the findings?

7. Explain how comparative data from similar hospitals in other metropolitan areas might be of use in interpreting the data.

Analysis and Interpretation

1. These data are attributes data because you know how many people completed the survey for each hospital and the number who marked excellent.

2. The data are binominally distributed, that is, we know both the occurrences and nonoccurrences of the "excellent" responses at each hospital. The proportion of "excellent" responses can be viewed as the proportion of "nondefective" responses. The u-chart would be used to show the rate of "total defects." For example, if several questions had been asked and we calculated the total number of "not-excellent" responses per patient.

3. The UCL and LCL are uneven because the number of patients responding varied considerably at each of the seven hospitals. Your hospital (#4) had the widest control limits because it had the fewest number of respondents (351 patients). Hospital 1 had the narrowest control limits because it had the highest number of respondents (1,426 patients). Given the wide differences in response rates among the seven hospitals, the stair-step approach to developing the control limits is appropriate.

4. There are no lines connecting the ratings of the seven hospitals because the control chart is not being used in this instance to compare a single hospital over a period of time,

but rather to compare seven different hospitals during the same time period.

5. It is possible, but highly unlikely, that the data from these seven hospitals are comparable. Before proceeding to analyze and interpret the p-chart, a number of questions need to be answered. In which way do the hospitals differ? Are they teaching hospitals or community hospitals? Are some city hospitals and other suburban hospitals? In which way do the patients differ? Is there an equal percentage of medical, surgical, and obstetric-gynecological patients at each hospital? What sampling method was used to conduct the survey? What was the overall response rate to the survey? Did the response rate differ considerably from one hospital to another? What safeguards were employed to reduce the interviewer bias normally associated with a phone survey?

6. In the unlikely event that the answers to questions 1 to 5 showed that the data from the seven hospitals were reasonably comparable, one might proceed to interpret the p-chart. Given the comparability of the data, one could conclude that only one hospital (hospital 7 with a 64 percent "excellent" rating) was a special cause and therefore different from the other hospitals. Although your hospital (4) received a 51 percent "excellent" rating, it is not appreciably different from the other five hospitals that are within the upper and lower control limits.

7. If it were possible to obtain comparable reference data from similar hospitals in other metropolitan areas, this would be of use in putting the data from your area into perspective. If the average percentage responding "excellent" on overall quality from other metropolitan areas was 45 percent, this would suggest that all seven hospitals in your metropolitan area were providing a relatively high level of quality care as perceived by patients. If comparable data from other metropolitan areas showed that the average percentage "excellent" was 70 percent, this would paint an entirely

different picture of patient satisfaction in your area. Comparable reference data to use as a "benchmark" are usually not readily available. However, some survey firms are beginning to build databases to provide such data.

Management Considerations

Developing a "report card" to measure patient satisfaction is a questionable procedure given the current state of the art. Conducting valid and reliable surveys requires professional planning, execution, and analysis. Many factors can bias the data and impede comparability. Nevertheless, numerous patient satisfaction report cards, such as the one described in this case study, have been developed. It is anticipated that this practice will continue to gain in popularity. Managers must be prepared, therefore, to deal with the potentially harmful publicity that can be caused by inappropriate comparisons or ranking of hospitals.

Finally, this case study is not meant to discourage the reader from using surveys in CQI. When properly conducted, surveys can be useful in identifying opportunities for improvement, in prioritizing opportunities for improvement, and in evaluating the degree of success of selected interventions. (See Chapter 8 for a discussion of the appropriate use of surveys in CQI efforts and the possible pitfalls in survey research.)

CASE STUDY 10: PATIENT FALLS

The Situation

In September 1991, your hospital introduced a new program to reduce the number of patient falls. As risk manager, you have been asked repeatedly, "Did this new program have the desired impact?" To determine the answer, you decide to take advantage of the knowledge and experience of the team that created the program. They have been working on this since January 1991 and have (1) developed and maintained a consistent operational definition of a patient fall (i.e., "an unplanned and unexpected change in a patient's position, with the patient landing on the floor"), (2) developed and implemented an ongoing data collection plan, and (3) prepared two control charts (found in Figures 6.17 and 6.18).

Figure 6.17 presents data for the 24 months from January 1, 1991, through December 31, 1992. During these months the census was relatively constant. Each data point represents the total number of falls occurring within all 20 units each month. Since the new prevention program was implemented in September 1991, Figure 6.17 shows the number of falls both before and after the prevention program. Note that the mean and control limits in this figure are based on the 9 months from January to September 1991, not on all 24 data points. Figure 6.18, on the other hand, shows data only for the 15 months following the introduction of the falls prevention program.

The Questions

1. Are patient falls to be considered attributes or variables data?

2. A c-chart was used to analyze the data. Is this type of chart appropriate? If it is not appropriate, what led you to this conclusion?

3. What would you have predicted after September 1991 regarding the number of patient falls if the falls prevention program had not been implemented?

4. Was the prevention program effective? How do you know? What tests to identify special causes were violated?

5. Why were the mean and the control limits in Figure 6.17 "frozen" after September 1991?

6. What new information is provided by the second control chart (Figure 6.18)?

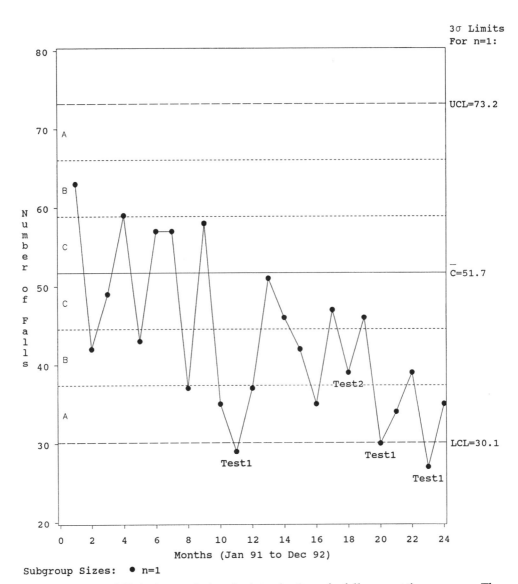

FIGURE 6.17. Inpatient falls before and after the introduction of a falls prevention program. The prevention program was introduced in September 1991 (month 9). The control limits are based on months 1 through 9.

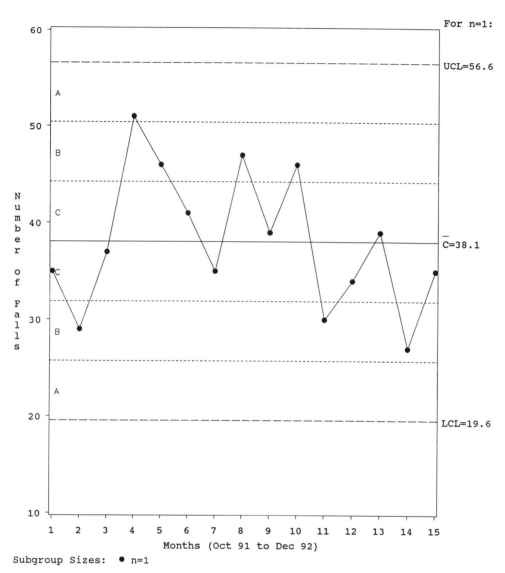

FIGURE 6.18. Inpatient falls after the introduction of a falls prevention program.

7. Does the second chart (Figure 6.18) show you whether the fall prevention process has improved sufficiently? If your team continues its efforts, how will you know whether these future efforts can be judged as successful?

Analysis and Interpretation

1. The number of patient falls should be considered attributes data. A fall can be considered as "defect" and you are counting the number of "defects" per month.

2. You will choose either a u-chart or a c-chart, because you do not know the number of non-occurrences or "non-falls." You do not know the number of "non-falls" because a patient might fall several times in the same day.

   The choice between a u-chart and a c-chart depends on whether there was an equal opportunity for patient falls to occur each month. If there had been considerable variation in the census from month to month during the years 1991 to 1992, you would have had to use a u-chart displaying the ratio of patient falls to total patient days. However, because you are considering all 20 units of your hospital taken together and the census during these months was relatively constant, a c-chart is also acceptable for this analysis. The c-chart was selected in this case because it has the advantage of enabling you to focus on the *actual number* of patient falls (as compared to *rate* of falls used in the u-chart).

3. If nothing had been done to address the number of patient falls during September 1991, the upper portion of Figure 6.17 shows what you would have expected to see, on the average about 52 falls per month. The upper and lower control limits show that during any given month, there might be as few as 30 falls or as many as 73 falls. The mean and control limits describe the process capability.

4. The control chart of Figure 6.17 shows that the fall prevention program was indeed effective. The data show that after the introduction of the prevention program, there were 8 consecutive months during which the average number of falls fell below the previous mean of 51.7 (indicated by the Test 2 violation printed on the chart). In addition, during 3 months after the introduction of the program, the number of falls fell beneath the lower control limit (indicated by a Test 1 violation). The results clearly show that there has been a shift in your process that produces falls.

5. The mean and limits were frozen after September 1991, because this was the month during which you introduced the fall prevention program. It is important to note that the data before and after the program can be compared only if the operational definition of a patient fall was the same over the entire period of time. If the operational definition of patient fall had been changed when the program was introduced, the analysis shown on these charts would be incorrect.

6. The second control chart (Figure 6.18) was constructed solely with the data from October 1991 through December 1992, the period after the introduction of the fall prevention program. The mean and control limits describe the current capability of the current fall prevention process. The capability of this process can be described by the mean (38.1 falls per month) and the upper and lower control limits (56.6 falls and 19.6 falls, respectively).

7. The information presented on these two control charts does not tell your team whether or not you should continue your efforts to reduce the number of patient falls. They merely tell your team that the initial efforts have been successful, and that your current process is characterized by about 38 falls per month, plus or minus approximately 19 falls per month. Should your team decide to introduce another intervention to further reduce the number of falls, it

will be able to judge that it has been successful if a test for a special cause is subsequently violated. For example, if during the next 8 months, the number of falls per month is less than the current process mean of 38.9 falls per month shown on Figure 6.18, then this would signal the success of your intervention. The new intervention could also be considered effective if the variation were decreased, that is, if the control limits were narrowed.

Management Considerations

To assist the team determine whether or not it should continue to work on patient falls, the team might use a Pareto diagram to investigate whether one or more units has a disproportionate number of patient falls. If one or more units are responsible for a large percentage of the falls each month, subsequent efforts to reduce falls could be focused on these units. In addition, the team might invite selected members of the staff from these units to become members of the falls prevention team.

The team would also be well advised to monitor the number of patient falls over the coming months, even if it decides not to introduce any other prevention efforts. The reason is that the team should want to be certain that the observed improvement is maintained during future months. Some employees may tend to focus less on falls once they know that the number of patient falls is no longer being monitored. New employees may also need to be trained in the details of the successful falls prevention program.

CASE 11: USE OF RESTRAINTS WITH PSYCHIATRIC PATIENTS

The Situation

How do you know whether the psychiatrists at your hospital are using restraints on patients too often? As the chairperson of the department of psychiatry quality assurance committee, you have had to respond to this question. Some of the nurses in the psychiatric units have even reported their concerns to your committee. Their specific concerns have been focused on the psychiatrists who joined the medical staff in 1992. The nurses suggest that the committee should either change the policy regarding restraints or talk to the psychiatrists regarding the increased use of restraints.

Your committee decided to develop the u-chart shown in Figure 6.19 to investigate whether current use of restraints offers an opportunity for improvement. Because some patients might be put in restraints two or three times a day, the committee decided to plot the monthly rate obtained by dividing the number of times restraints were recorded in the patient charts by the number of total patient days.

After viewing the chart, the committee decided to investigate why the rate was high for months 13 to 15 (January to March 1992). They found that the increased use was due to one seriously disturbed patient who had been put in restraints two to three times per day during this 3-month period before he was discharged. In the view of the committee, the restraints were appropriately used for this patient. Therefore, the committee decided to generate another chart (Figure 6.20) after removing the data regarding the seriously disturbed patient.

The Questions

1. Are the rates plotted on the charts considered variables or attributes data?

2. Is the u-chart appropriate? Why did the committee not use a c-chart or perhaps a p-chart?

3. Does Figure 6.19 show that the restraint process is in control? If it is not in control, what test(s) to identify special cause(s) is applicable?

4. What can the committee predict regarding the process of utilizing restraints?

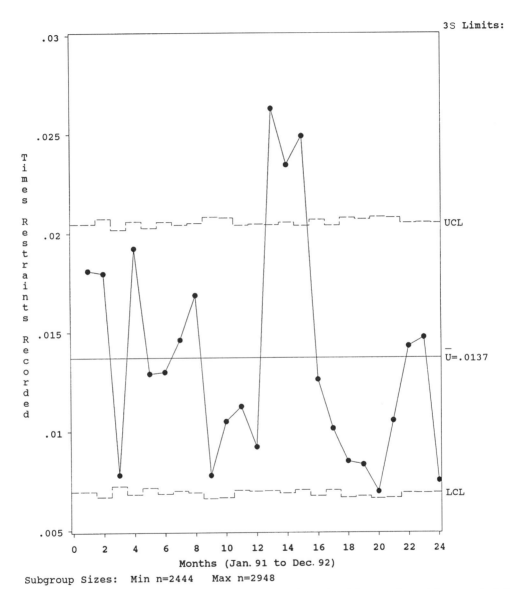

FIGURE 6.19. Use of restraints with psychiatric patients (the ratio of the number of times restraints recorded to the patient days per month).

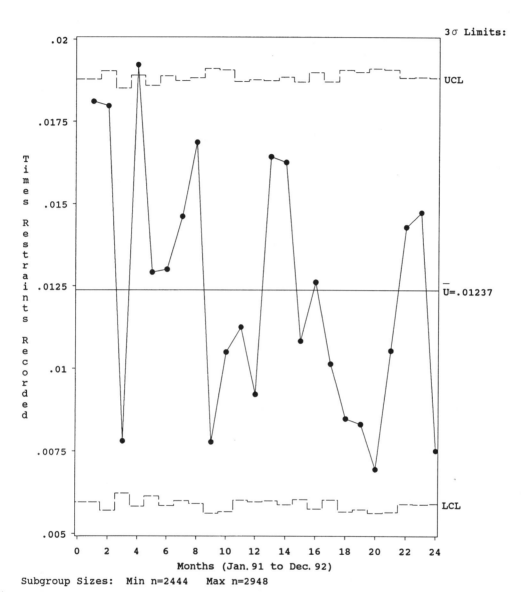

FIGURE 6.20. Follow up: Use of restraints with psychiatric patients (the ratio of the number of times restraints recorded to the patient days per month after removing data from the seriously disturbed patient who was properly restrained from months 13 to 15).

5. Did the committee act appropriately in removing the seriously disturbed patient from the database and generating a new chart? Why or why not?

6. What did the second u-chart (Figure 6.20) tell the committee?

7. What should the committee do next? Should it modify the restraint policy based on these charts?

Analysis and Interpretation

1. The data recording the use of patient restraints is properly considered attributes data because the committee is counting the use of restraints as "defects."

2. The u-chart is the correct chart because the number of patient days varied from month to month, thereby creating an unequal area of opportunity for defects to occur. The committee would not use a p-chart unless it was analyzing the percentage of patients who were put in restraints each month, but did not feel it was important to determine whether restraints were used one or more times for each patient.

3. The process is not in control. The data from months 13 to 15 (January to March 1992) were far beyond the upper control limit.

4. The committee cannot predict what to expect from its restraint process in the future, because the restraint process is not in control, that is, one or more special causes were present. This makes the process unstable and unpredictable.

5. The committee determined that the origin of the special cause was a particularly troubled and violent patient who had to be restrained several times a day, not the restraint process itself. Therefore, the committee was correct when it

removed the data for this patient and recalculated the control limits.

6. The second control chart (Figure 6.20) showed the committee that the new psychiatrists admitted to the staff in 1992 had not been overusing restraints as compared to the practice of the staff in 1991. However, the process is still not in control because another special cause (previously hidden by the first set of special causes) was identified in month 4 (April 1991). Therefore, the committee still cannot accurately predict the capability of the restraint process.

7. If time and resources permit, the committee should examine the patient charts for April 1991 to determine the origin of the special cause that was previously hidden in the first control chart (Figure 6.19). However, because almost 2 years have passed since this special cause occurred, and because the data have been in control for the past 20 months, the committee might be justified in choosing to examine the data for the past 20 months, and in asking whether the observed rate (approximately 12 patients put in restraints for every 1,000 patient days) is an appropriate frequency considering the severity of patients currently being treated. If the committee decides that this frequency is appropriate, then it might choose to pursue a different opportunity for quality improvement.

Management Considerations

In this example, the nurses apparently remembered the increased use of restraints during the months of January to March 1992, and generalized from this memory to characterize the practice during the rest of 1992. However, analysis of the data showed that, with the exception of a single patient, the use of restraints had not increased since the new psychiatrists joined the medical staff in 1992. A control chart helped to correct their impressions.

This example also shows that one special cause can be hidden by another special cause. Even after the committee was able to identify the origin of the special cause in months 13 and 15, it still could not accurately predict the process capability from the data in the second control chart due to another special cause. Nevertheless, it might be difficult to justify spending the time and energy to identify a special cause in data that are nearly 2 years old.

CASE STUDY 12: MEDICATION ERRORS

The Situation

As vice president in charge of patient care services, one of your areas of responsibilities is the pharmacy department. Nine weeks ago you hired a new director of the pharmacy. The director has presented you with a line chart showing a decrease in the medication error rate from approximately 5.2 errors per 10,000 orders to 2.3 per 10,000 orders since he arrived (Figure 6.21). He believes that he deserves special recognition because the number of medication errors since the time he was hired has been "significantly" reduced.

The director has operationally defined "medication errors" as being any one of the following: the wrong medication; the wrong dose; administered at the wrong time; administered to the wrong patient; incorrectly repeating the medication; or omitting the medication. Currently, the pharmacy is filling approximately 25,000 to 32,000 orders per week. The number of medication errors has ranged from 4 to 15 errors per week. More than one error might occur on the same medication order.

Subsequent to your new director's request, you have asked your CQI statistician to develop a control chart that would enable you to analyze medication error rates, both before and after the arrival of the new pharmacy director. The statistician has given you a u-chart with data for 11 weeks prior to the arrival of the new director and for 9 weeks after his arrival (Figure 6.22).

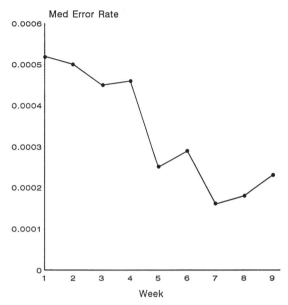

FIGURE 6.21. Medication error rate for the new director. Error rate = number of errors/total orders per week.

The Questions

1. What type of data are medication errors?

2. Why did the statistician choose to make a u-chart rather than a c-chart?

3. Was the upward pattern in the medication errors observed during the previous director's tenure a special cause? Was the "improvement" under the new director's management a special cause?

4. On the basis of these data, do you believe the number of medication errors has been "significantly" reduced? Why or why not?

5. What medication error rate can be expected under the current process?

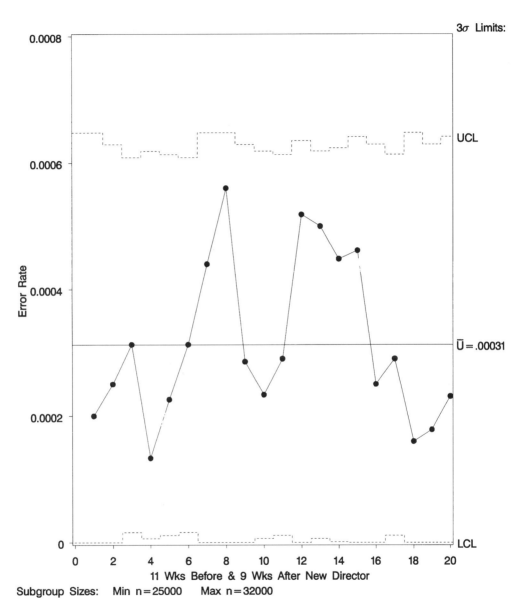

FIGURE 6.22. Medication error rate for the past 20 weeks (11 weeks before and 9 weeks after arrival of the new director). Error rate = number of errors/total orders per week.

6. What would your new director need to accomplish to show that his pharmacy team has achieved a downward shift in the medication error rate?

Analysis and Interpretation

1. Each medication error can be viewed as a defect and should be considered attributes data.

2. A u-chart rather than a c-chart is the appropriate choice because the area of opportunity for medication errors is unequal from week to week. (The number of medication orders processed varied from 25,000 to 32,000 per week.) If the statistician had chosen to take an equal random sample of orders from week to week, then he would have chosen to use a c-chart. A c-chart might also have been acceptable if the number of orders had only slight variation from week to week. A c-chart has the advantage of examining the actual number of errors rather than the rate of errors, and consequently is easier for some people to analyze and understand. A c-chart would also have permitted the use of zone tests for special causes in addition to the more common tests and would have produced straight-line control limits rather than stair-stepped limits.

3. What appeared to be a "upward trend" from the fourth to the eighth week under the old director was not a true statistical trend as defined by the tests for a special cause, which would require six ascending points (with less than 21 points) before the "trend" could be identified as a special cause. Furthermore, the data do not show a special cause after the arrival of the new director. The data for the last 5 weeks are indeed below the center line, but one would have to observe eight consecutive points below the mean before identifying a shift in the process that would constitute a special cause.

4. On the basis of these data, you cannot say that the number of medication errors has been significantly reduced. No tests for special causes are violated. Although there is a fair amount of variation, it is common-cause variation and the process is in control and predictable.

5. The current process capability can be defined by the mean and the upper and lower control limits. If no change takes place in the current process, one can expect to observe on the average about 3.1 errors per 10,000 medication orders with as many as 6.3 per 10,000 or as few as none in any given week. However, the control chart does not tell you whether the current rate is acceptable.

6. To show that his pharmacy team had indeed brought about a downward shift in the medication error rate, the new director should continue to plot the data for the coming weeks. If the next 3 weeks continue to show an error rate below the mean of 3.1 errors per 10,000 orders, this would produce a run of eight data points, signaling a special cause.

Management Considerations

A manager not acquainted with statistical process control theory might easily have seen an upward trend in errors before the new director's arrival and a downward trend since he began work at the hospital. However, the variability in both instances can best be viewed as "noise," not a "signal." It is an all too human failing for someone to take personal credit when a process appears to improve and to blame others when a process appears to deteriorate. Using the tests for special causes provides a more objective basis for making judgments about process performance.

7

Developing
Improvement Strategies

At this point, the patience of some readers may be strained. Some may well ask, "When are the authors going to describe some specific suggestions for improving the processes they presented in their case studies?" Alas, those readers are about to be disappointed! Run charts and control charts will not tell a quality improvement team how its process should be improved. Nor will control charts tell a team the reason for a special cause, nor whether a process with only common-cause variation should be improved. Only those who know the process are in a position to develop an improvement strategy for that particular process. However, it is a fair question to ask, "Now that I have collected data and constructed a run or control chart, what is next?"

The Type of Variation Determines Your Strategy

After you have completed the control chart, it is time to develop an improvement strategy. The approach will be determined by the source and type of variation on the chart. For example, if you observe a special cause, you will want to investigate its origin. If the special cause is a negative or undesirable factor, you will try to eliminate the factors that produce this deviation in your process.

If it is a positive event, you will still want to investigate the special cause, determine if you can emulate it, and make it a standard part of the process.

If on the other hand, you observe only common-cause variation, your quality improvement team must decide whether the process average and upper and lower control limits, which define process capability, suggest that the process should be improved. If appropriate benchmark data are available, these data can be used to assist in making this judgment. The customer served by your process may also help you decide whether to improve the process.

If your team decides to try to improve a common-cause process, they can accomplish this by (1) reducing the amount of variation (i.e., by narrowing the width of the control limits) and/or (2) moving the process average in the desired direction. Note that improvement is accomplished by one or both of these actions.

Right and Wrong Strategies

Figure 7.1 describes the appropriate and inappropriate management approaches to special- and common-cause variation. If your process has both special- and common-cause variation, the wrong choice will be to change the process in reaction to an undesired special cause. The right strategy is to investigate the special cause and remove it. For example, in 1992, large amounts of medical waste material, such as syringes, vials, bloody gauze, began to wash up on the beaches of New York and New Jersey. In response to the public outcry for action, the Environmental Protection Agency responded by forcing hospitals in those states to place a wide range of designated waste products in red bags and dispose of the waste with special handling. To avoid severe penalties, hospitals began to "red bag" most waste, thereby adding millions of dollars in cost to hospital expenses. However, the real origin of the problem was not the hospitals, but disposal companies that tried to save money by having their waste barges dump hospital waste too close to the shoreline. An inappropriate management response

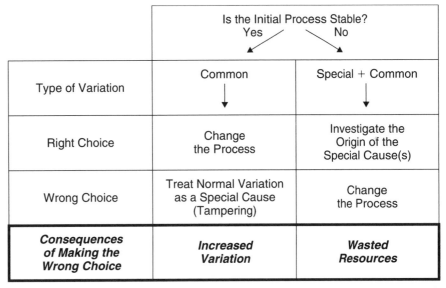

FIGURE 7.1. **Appropriate management response to common and special causes of variation.**

to the problem (changing the hospital disposal process) resulted in wasted resources. The appropriate response would have been to identify the origin of the special cause (the dumping by waste barges) and eliminate it.

Or consider another example of a situation in a hospital where thousands of operations had been performed without a surgeon ever leaving a sponge inside a patient. However, on one occasion when a sponge was left inside a patient, the patient sued the hospital and the board of trustees demanded that the medical staff take immediate action. The medical staff responded by changing the operating procedure so that after every abdominal surgery, the patient would have to be x-rayed before leaving the operating room. This change resulted in needlessly exposing patients to radiation and increasing the cost of all abdominal operations. The correct management response would have been to identify the source of the special cause and take steps to prevent it from happening again.

Figure 7.1 also shows that if a process displays only common-cause variation, the wrong management approach is to treat every occurrence as a special cause. Deming (1986: 54) gives an example of this error. A supervisor was known for her great patience and compassion because she would spend the last half-hour of every day working with her seven employees examining and scrutinizing every defective item. Everyone thought she was a great supervisor, but the fact was that the system was stable, and the observed defects were part of a common-cause system. The people were not at fault; the system was. The supervisor was treating every fault and blemish as a special cause, instead of trying to improve the system.

Changing a Common-Cause System

Let us suppose that your team has plotted data on a control chart and the data revealed only common-cause variation. After discussion with your customer, your team decides that the process should be improved. What are the next steps?

Figure 7.2 is the same process improvement road map that you saw back in Chapter 1. Beneath the diamond that contains the question, "Are special causes present?" you will observe the next steps to be taken if the answer is "no." If you decide your process should be improved, you first identify process variables (PVs) or those aspects or factors of a process that potentially have an impact on the key quality characteristic (KQC).

Next, you choose from among the process variables one that you think might have the largest impact on the variation you observed on your control chart. This variable, which we can call a key process variable (KPV), will become the focal point of your efforts to improve the key quality characteristic of your process. For example, suppose that you are the director of the laboratory and that your team had chosen "promptness" as a KQC of your process. Key process variables that might influence promptness or turnaround time might include (1) the log-in procedure in the lab; (2) the pickup and delivery schedule; (3) staffing; and (4) the pneumatic tube system. From these four items, you might decide to focus on the tube system as the first KPV that you wish to in-

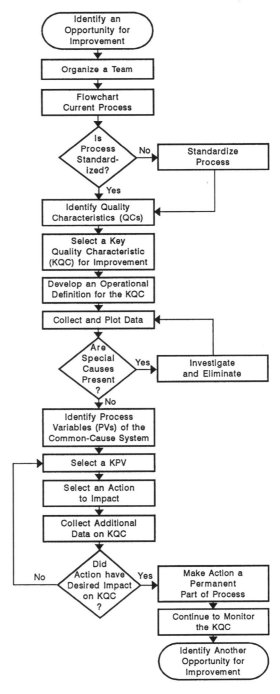

FIGURE 7.2. Process improvement flowchart.

vestigate.

After selecting a KPV, you would identify actions that you believe might have a major impact on the KPV. From these actions, you would select an action to implement. In the case of the lab example, an action might be to order more containers for the tube system.

Finally, you would proceed to collect additional data on turnaround time (the KQC) and observe whether the action you implemented had the desired impact. If a special cause appears on the chart in the desired direction, then you will know that your action had the desired impact and you will make this action (having an adequate number of containers available) a permanent part of the process. If the data did not show a special cause in the desired direction (i.e., a decreased turnaround time), then you would select a different action or different KPV and once again collect more data on the KQC.

Figure 7.3 graphs the relationship between the KQC and the KPVs described before by showing that the KQC may be influenced by more than one KPV, and that each KPV might have more than one action associated with it.

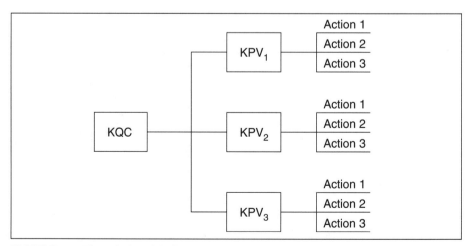

FIGURE 7.3. **The relationship between a KQC and its KPVs.**

Figure 7.4 is a heuristic diagram to illustrate how an improvement strategy might work successfully to reduce the number of late lab tests. In this example, the number of late lab tests would be noted on the left margin. An initial investigation (Time 1) showed that the average of late tests for 17 consecutive days was unacceptable and also that there was wide variations from day to day. Next, because the improvement team discovered that the delivery process was different on the day and evening shifts, they agreed to standardize the process before trying to make other changes (Time 2). The standardization had the effect of both reducing variation and decreasing the number of late tests to some extent. Then the team introduced an action to affect the first KPV (Time 3), perhaps a change in the tube system as described before, with the result of a decrease in the number of late tests. Finally, the team introduced an action to affect second KPV, perhaps hiring an additional bench technician in the lab. Additional data were collected (Time 4), ideally resulting in continued improvement.

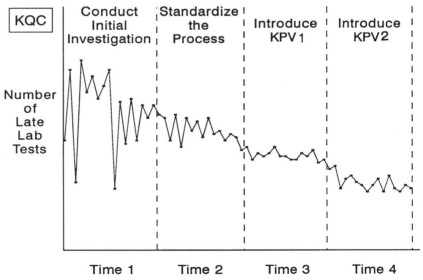

FIGURE 7.4. KQC improvement strategy.

Tools to Identify KPVs

Pareto Diagrams

In Chapter 2, the use of a Pareto diagram for identifying and prioritizing key quality characteristics was discussed. An example was given of the use of a Pareto diagram to prioritize patient complaints identified through a patient survey. The Pareto diagram enabled the quality improvement team to separate the "vital few" complaints that were most likely to contribute to patient dissatisfaction, thereby enabling time and resources to be used where they would have the best payoff.

The Pareto diagram also can be used later in the quality improvement process to choose a key process variable from among many potential process variables. For example, suppose that you are the director of the pharmacy department and wished to reduce medication errors. First, you analyzed the total number of medication errors over the last 13 months. By stratifying the data, you observed that although there was an average of 40 errors per month, 23 were intravenous (IV) administration errors and only 17 were non-IV errors. Therefore, to lower the total number of errors you decided to concentrate first on IV errors.

Next, to check on whether the process for delivering IV medications was stable, you used the c-chart (Figure 7.5) to analyze the data. (You used a c-chart because you were considering medication errors as "defects" and the number of IV orders varied only slightly each month.) The c-chart showed that your process was in control and therefore it would be an appropriate candidate for a process improvement strategy.

But where should you begin? You heard many complaints from your staff pharmacists that physicians were ordering IV medications inappropriately. These were written up in "occurrence reports" as "prescribing concerns." However, you decided to examine the number of the "prescribing concerns" along with the other most common IV medication errors and to analyze them

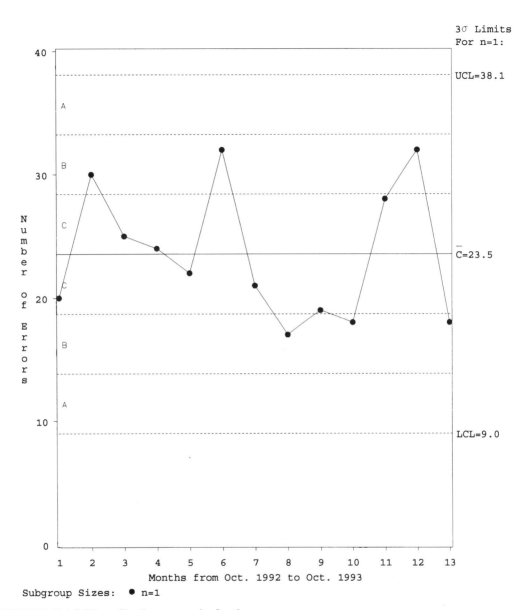

FIGURE 7.5. Total IV medication errors (c-chart).

using a Pareto diagram. Figure 7.6 shows that of 282 IV errors, the most common was giving the wrong dose (104, or 37%). Omitting the dose accounted for 66 (23%), and the wrong solution accounted for 63 (22%). Together, these three problems accounted for 82% of all IV medication errors. By analyzing the Pareto diagram in Figure 7.6, it was easy to see that by focusing on "wrong dose," you would have the best chance of reducing the total number of IV errors.

Next, you plotted the monthly number of wrong-dose IV medication errors for the same 13 months (Figure 7.7). You can see immediately that this process has a special cause (month 2 is outside the upper control limit). Now the team must address the special cause detected by this control chart. Without having used a Pareto

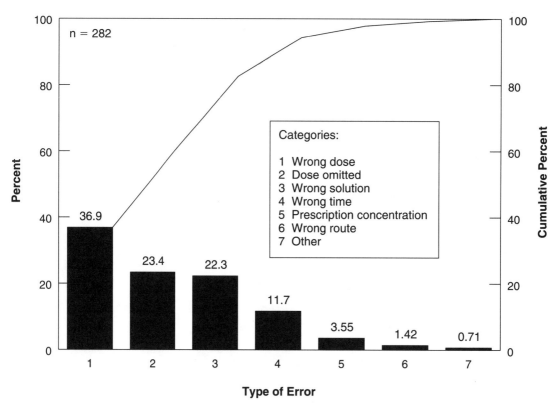

FIGURE 7.6. Type of IV medication errors (total number of errors from October 1992 to October 1993).

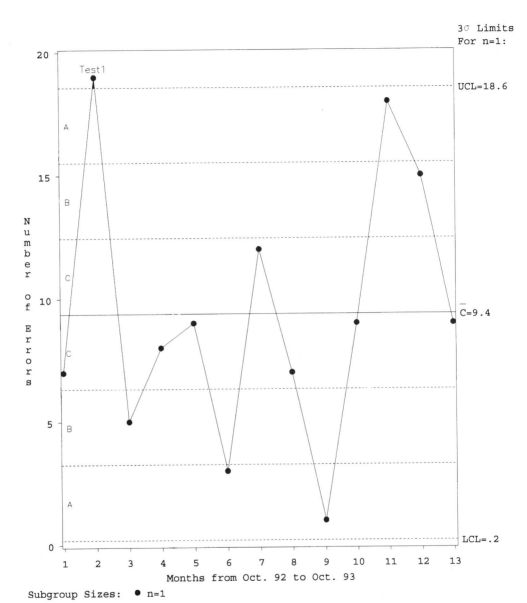

FIGURE 7.7. IV medication errors: incorrect dose (c-chart).

diagram, the team would not have identified the major contributor to medication errors.

Cause-and-Effect Diagrams

Another tool to help select a key process variable from among many possible process variables is the cause-and-effect diagram, also known as the Ishikawa diagram or a fishbone diagram. The "effect" is the problem, issue, or event being studied—in other words, the key quality characteristic. The effect is placed in a box at the right-hand side of the page. Then a horizontal line is drawn to the left of the effect. Diagonal lines are drawn above and below the horizontal line. These "branches" are titled with categories of "causes." Frequently used categories are people, methods, materials, equipment, and environment.

The purpose of the cause-and-effect diagram is to facilitate discussion by the quality improvement team. It forces people to think explicitly about the specifics of the process, as well as about their customers and suppliers. A more complete explanation of the construction and use of this tool can be found in Ishikawa (1982: Chapter 3).

An illustration of the cause-and-effect diagram is provided in Figure 7.8. The reader may wish to refer to Case Study 6 in Chapter 6, which described the use of an XmR chart to analyze the transfer process of a patient from the emergency department to an inpatient room. You will recall that the total transfer time was divided into two parts (from the time the ER called the admitting department to the time the bed was assigned, and from the time when the bed was assigned until the patient arrived in the room on the unit). The second part of this process required most of the total time. This part of the process was also in control. Therefore, it was appropriate for the team to try to improve this process.

Figure 7.8 illustrates how the team might use a cause-and-effect diagram to identify the possible process variables that affect transfer time. The key quality characteristic (timeliness of the

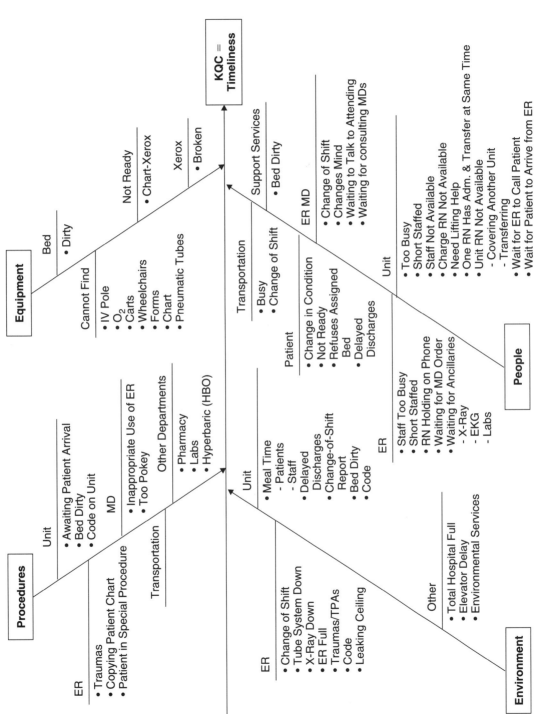

FIGURE 7.8. ER bed transfer cause-and-effect diagram.

transfer) is placed in the box at the right margin. Then the team used four major categories to group the process variables: procedures, equipment, environment, and people.

One observation became clear very quickly. Placing the major portion of the problem of delay on the shoulders of the transportation personnel would be oversimplifying the factors that contribute to creating delays in the bed transfer process.

Continued Monitoring

Returning again to Figure 7.2, notice that even if the action you chose had the desired impact on the KQC and was made a permanent part of the process, you would want to continue to monitor the KQC, at least periodically, to ensure that the improvement continues. This is especially true when the KPV involves changing people's behavior. It is not uncommon, for example, for people to perform better when they know that their actions are being monitored, and then return to their old ways after monitoring is completed. Those of you who have reduced the speed of your automobile because you observe the police clearly understand this principle.

How Much Improvement Is Enough?

When should a team stop trying to improve a process and turn its efforts to another opportunity for improvement? This is a question for each team to decide. The decision will be influenced by a number of factors: (1) customer priorities; (2) the relative impact of a process on patient care and cost; (3) the amount of resources (i.e., staff and money) available; and (4) the level of the team's enthusiasm. Identifying opportunities for improvement is usually not as difficult as selecting the one that will have the biggest payoff for the team and its customers.

8

Using Patient Surveys for CQI

For decades, healthcare providers have used patient surveys to gain a better understanding of how they are perceived. Starting in the late 1980s, however, patient surveys began to play a more prominent role in determining the "quality" of delivered care. For example, "report cards" of care developed by many managed care plans, such as United HealthCare Corporation in Minneapolis, the Cleveland Health Quality Choice Coalition, and Kaiser Permanente in California have included surveys of customer satisfaction among the indicators of quality. In addition, many hospitals and healthcare systems have made widespread use of patient surveys to focus quality improvement efforts and to measure the results of interventions.

Survey questionnaires have not always been developed and analyzed with adequate attention to the principles of survey research. Many hospitals and healthcare facilities, for example, develop their own in-house surveys without receiving any input from those skilled in the design and analysis of surveys. In addition, individual nursing units and various departmental providers within hospitals, such as physical therapy, occupational therapy, and respiratory therapy, add to the proliferation of surveys by developing their own instruments for patients treated in their areas. On the other hand, some facilities recognizing the limitations of well-intentioned, amateur efforts have hired commercial survey firms, but without adequately assessing the quality of the reports they receive from these firms.

The growing proliferation of surveys is due in part to the feeling that conducting patient surveys is a simple process. Popular opinion seems to be that all one needs to do is to develop a series of questions, interview a number of patients by phone or mail, and tally the results. However, the path of survey research has hidden pitfalls and land mines. Therefore, those who do not wish to risk serious misjudgments should use surveys with the proper care and attention to the principles of survey research.

A Self-Test on Survey Research

If you are using patient surveys either for the purpose of developing report cards or for CQI, you should be able to comfortably address the following nine questions:

1. What is the role or function of patient surveys in CQI efforts? Are they best used as enumerative studies or analytic studies? Should they be used to measure the voice of the customer or to measure the voice of the process?

2. What is the meaning of a "reliable" survey questionnaire? A "valid" questionnaire?

3. Why is reliability important?

4. How do you know whether your survey has adequate reliability?

5. How do you know you are using an appropriate sampling method for your survey? Are you able to estimate your sampling error?

6. How are you controlling for the problem of biased data? Interviewer bias? Response bias?

7. Are you communicating survey results effectively? Do managers use the reports? What types of statistical analyses are appropriate for survey data?

8. Do you use benchmark data (or comparative reference data) to assist your managers interpret the findings? What is the quality of your benchmark data?

9. How are you using survey data to evaluate the effectiveness of management interventions?

If you had difficulty answering these questions, you will find this chapter useful. This chapter makes no attempt to teach the reader how to construct or execute surveys, but only to identify and explain the key issues with which you should be concerned.

Function of Patient Surveys in CQI

A periodic patient survey (perhaps done on a quarterly basis) is perhaps best used as an enumerative study to measure the voice of the customer. First, surveys can identify opportunities for improvement. Second, this information can be used to set priorities among the identified opportunities (by using a Pareto diagram). In this way, surveys can guide the focus of analytic studies that measure the voice of the process. Then, after the completion of an analytic study, a follow-up survey can be conducted to measure the extent to which the improvement observed in an analytic study has been perceived by the customer.

It will be helpful for the reader to recall at this time the difference between enumerative and analytic studies described in Chapter 3. By an enumerative study, we mean a study that is done on a static population for a given time period to describe some outcome of interest. It might be compared to taking a snapshot of a group of patients. An enumerative study answers such questions as: "What was the average length of stay for patients last year? What was the percentage of surgical patients admitted last year?"

An analytic study, on the other hand, is one that is done on a dynamic process, is not restricted to a single point in time, and is used to predict the future rather than describe past outcomes. In this respect, an analytic study can be compared to a video recording rather than to a snapshot. Analytic studies are done to determine *why* the outcomes were observed and *how* the process that produced the outcomes can be improved. An analytic study answers questions such as: "What can we predict about the length of stay for the coming year? What were the causes of the observed decrease in surgical inpatients for the previous year?" A more extensive overview of the differences between enumerative and analytic studies can be found in Gitlow et al. (1989).

Figure 8.1 is a heuristic diagram that illustrates how an enumerative survey of emergency room (ER) patients might be used as part of a CQI effort to reduce waiting time. At Time 1, this hospital conducted a survey of ER patients to determine their degree of satisfaction with various aspects of patient care, such as waiting time, explanation of diagnosis and treatment, adequacy of discharge instructions, and so forth. Suppose that the results of the survey showed that waiting time was the issue with which patients were

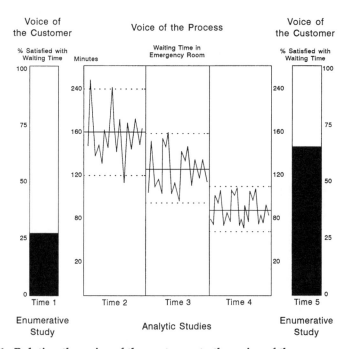

FIGURE 8.1. **Relating the voice of the customer to the voice of the process.**

least satisfied (only 25% were satisfied) and that the majority wanted to be treated and discharged in less than 2 hours. As a result of this enumerative study, the CQI team in the ER decided to measure the voice of the process by conducting an analytic study of actual waiting time. Figure 8.1 shows that during Time 2, the actual waiting times for 25 consecutive patients were recorded and plotted on an XmR chart. Results show that the average waiting time was 160 minutes (2.7 hours) and that the process showed wide variation with some waiting times both above and below the control limits.

Next, the CQI team developed an intervention (the exact details of which are unimportant for this illustration) and collected data on 25 more patients during Time 3 (Figure 8.1). Results showed that the average wait time was reduced to a little over 2 hours and the degree of variation was also reduced. However, the improvement was still not up to customer expectations (i.e., less than 2 hours). Therefore, another intervention was introduced and data were collected on 25 more patients during Time 4. Results for this period now showed that the average wait time was reduced to approximately 85 minutes and the upper control limit was now below the 2-hour time limit voiced by patients in the enumerative study conducted during Time 1.

Finally, during Time 5, the same patient questionnaire used during Time 1 was repeated. Results showed that the percentage of patients satisfied with the waiting time had increased substantially to approximately 70 percent. The analytic study used to measure the voice of the process showed that there had been two dramatic shifts in the process from Time 2 to Time 3 and from Time 3 to Time 4. The enumerative study (a patient survey) at Time 5 showed the extent to which this improvement had been perceived by patients.

We are not saying that surveys are the only way to *listen* to the voice of the customer, or to identify opportunities for improvement. A CQI team also can use focus groups, complaint letters, customer defection, or personal observation in the ER to identify that waiting time is a problem. However, we are saying that surveys are the best tools to *measure* the voice of the customer and especially to evaluate the amount of *perceived* progress achieved by an analytic study.

Nor is it the position of the authors that patient survey data cannot be used in an analytic study to determine the effectiveness of intervention programs. Hayes (1992) has described how customer satisfaction data can be used to evaluate interventions using control charts. He describes how to develop a customer satisfaction questionnaire that has reliability and validity, and then how $\overline{X}$-S charts, p-charts, and c-charts can be used to analyze survey data from customers of service organizations. However, whereas Hayes emphasizes the critical importance of having a questionnaire with demonstrated reliability and validity, his control chart examples assume the existence of adequate sampling, representative response rate, and sufficient data points to compute stable control limits.

We would agree with Hayes that patient survey data indeed can be used in an analytic study if all the previous assumptions are verified. However, it is our feeling that most healthcare facilities do not have the expertise and logistic support to conduct analytic studies in the manner described by Hayes. Analyzing patient survey data with control charts as part of an analytic study is considerably more difficult than analyzing surveys of banking customers (in Hayes' illustration). The sampling methodology is more complicated, avoiding interviewer bias is more difficult, collecting adequate data in a timely manner with a good response rate is more costly, and selecting the appropriate control chart is not always straightforward. Therefore, we recommend that most hospitals and healthcare providers initially use patient surveys as enumerative studies, as described earlier.

Reliability and Validity

Because no patient questionnaire will ever assess patient satisfaction with perfect accuracy, we will never know the true level of patient satisfaction. Therefore, we need to assess the degree of accuracy of a questionnaire by measuring its reliability. Reliability as we are using it in the present context refers to how well ratings obtained by a questionnaire reflect actual levels of patient satisfaction on a particular dimension of patient experience (such as nursing care, physician care, or housekeeping service). Reliability in this sense is called internal consistency to distinguish it from other types of reliability (such as test–retest reliability).

To assess patient opinion on a particular dimension of patient experience (e.g., nursing care), one might use a single question ("How would you rate nursing care overall?") in an effort to keep a questionnaire as brief as possible. Or one might ask several questions regarding various aspects of nursing care, for example, how well nurses answered questions, how promptly they responded to the call button, their courtesy, and so forth. The use of two or more questions to describe a dimension of care is referred to as a "scale." Combining the ratings of individual questions that make up a scale is called a "scale score."

Because reliability measures the degree of interrelationship of items, it can only be estimated with scales that have more than one item. Therefore, people who use one-item measures to assess the level of satisfaction of nursing care, physician care, or other issues of interest run the risk of obtaining information that is not highly reliable, that is, one cannot tell the extent to which the observed score on the one-item measure is related to the true level of satisfaction. Many questionnaires developed by inexperienced surveyors suffer from this important failing.

There are several methods to estimate the degree of reliability. The most common method is the Cronbach (1951) alpha statistic. This statistic estimates a scale's homogeneity or its degree of internal consistency, that is, it will tell you how well the items in a given scale are interrelated. The higher the interrelationship between the items, the higher the reliability of the scale and the better the scale will reflect the true level of patient satisfaction with the particular dimension of patient experience under investigation.

Validity, on the other hand, refers to the degree to which a scale measures what it is designed to measure. Unlike mathematical indices of reliability, such as the Cronbach alpha, there is not one statistic that provides an overall index of validity of scale scores. Inexperienced surveyors will often be satisfied with face validity. For example, if several questions all include a reference to nurses, one might be inclined to say that the scale has face validity for measuring nursing care. However, if you wish to determine whether the scales you developed with the intention of measuring distinct and separate aspects of care are viewed in the same way by respondents, then you are asking whether the questionnaire has construct validity. Construct validity can be assessed by conducting a factor analysis (Harman, 1976), examining the resulting scale patterns, and then assessing scale independence by studying interscale correlations.

In addition to construct validity, scales can be said to have predictive validity to the extent to which there is a systematic relationship between the scores on a given scale and other scores that it should predict. For example, scales designed to measure nursing care, physician care, and medical outcomes should be able to explain a high proportion of a patient's evaluation of overall quality or their willingness to recommend a facility. Regression analysis is the method ordinarily used to measure predictive validity. (Regression analysis is explained more fully in standard statistical texts.)

Why Is Reliability Important?

There are two reasons for having a scale with high reliability. First, because reliability indicates the degree to which observed scores are related to true scores, scales with high reliability will enable you to better distinguish between respondents on a continuum of patient satisfaction. If you cannot accurately detect differences in satisfaction levels, then there is a danger that a successful CQI intervention may appear not to have improved the process. One might erroneously conclude that the intervention ended in failure, when indeed it actually improved a process. Or it is possible to conclude that an intervention had a positive impact, when in reality it did not. Second, high reliability makes it more likely that you will find a significant relationship between variables that are truly related to each other, for example, satisfaction with physician care and a patient's willingness to recommend a hospital. The predictive validity of a scale will appear to be less than it actually is if the scale has poor reliability.

How Much Reliability Is Enough?

There is no rigid rule to determine an acceptable level of reliability. Reliability levels can be evaluated according to the stage of instrument development and/or the intended use of the scale. Nunnally (1967) states that in the early phase of scale development modest reliabilities of .60 and .50 are sufficient. Another criterion offered by Helmstadter (1964) is whether a measure is intended to compare groups or to compare individuals. For the former comparison a reliability of .50 is considered acceptable, while a minimum reliability level of .90 is recommended for comparison of individuals. A more extensive discussion of this issue is beyond the scope of this book.

Let us summarize reliability and validity issues: The patient survey that you utilize should have multiple-item scales, because single-item scales do not allow you to estimate reliability. The reliability of your scales should be at least 0.50 as measured by the Cronbach alpha statistic. Although a satisfactory level of predictive validity is even more difficult to determine, a good survey should be able to explain at least half of the variance of patients' evaluation of overall quality or their willingness to recommend your facility. Those who wish a detailed illustration of how reliability and validity have been developed for patient surveys are referred to an article by Carey and Seibert (1993).

Sampling

In Chapter 3, the differences between simple random sampling, proportionate random sampling, and judgment sampling were discussed. Before collecting data, it is our suggestion that expert counsel be sought with respect to sampling. For example, if you plan to use your survey as an enumerative study, then you will very likely want to use proportionate random sampling (e.g., by nursing unit, by site, and so forth). If you plan to use a patient survey as an analytic study, then you will want to use judgment sampling (e.g., by taking a sample of 40 patients a week by nursing unit or by site for 16 to 25 weeks).

You also need to ask yourself whether the sample you have chosen is adequate for your planned analysis. For example, in an enumerative study, how certain do you wish to be of the observed differences among nursing units or between shifts in the ER? What amount of sampling error are your prepared to accept? If you are employing professional surveyors to assist you, it is appropriate to expect them to estimate and report the degree of sampling error in the reports they provide you. In this regard, you may have noticed that when newspapers report survey results, they usually provide the "margin of error" of ±3 or ±4 percentage points connected with the survey. This statistic tells you the level of sampling error you can expect.

Interviewer and Nonresponse Bias

In addition to using a poor sampling methodology, there are two other types of bias that affect survey data: (1) interviewer bias and (2) nonresponse bias.

Interviewer bias is often associated with personal interviews and telephone surveys. Interviewer bias occurs when the persons being interviewed overreact in a negative or positive way to the interviewer, with the result that they do not reveal their true feelings. For example, a patient who is interviewed by a nurse before being discharged regarding the quality of medical or nursing care may be reluctant to respond negatively for fear of being considered rude or confrontational. Or discharged patients contacted by telephone at home may be reluctant to answer questions about physician care for fear that their comments will be shared with their personal physician and possibly damage their future relationship with the physician. Interviewer bias can also result from irritation with the interviewer due to perceived gender, racial, or age differences.

Nonresponse bias is more typical of mailed surveys. Even assuming an appropriate sampling methodology, if one obtained responses of only 20 to 30 percent of the patients sampled, how representative will the data be of the entire population to which you wish to generalize your findings? There is no consensus on the percentage required for a representative response rate. Some researchers, such as Babbie (1989), argue that a 50 percent or better response rate is necessary to generalize from the data. Others require an even higher percentage. It is certainly safer to generalize from a majority to a minority than from a minority to the majority.

Although achieving a higher response rate is used as an argument for conducting telephone surveys instead of mailed surveys, telephone surveyors have been known to inflate their reported response rate by reporting what is known as the "cooperation rate" instead of the actual response rate. For example, if you mail questionnaires to a sample of 300 patients and obtain 180 returned questionnaires, your response rate is 60 percent. If you try to contact the same 300 people by phone and are able to contact only 200 patients of which 180 agree to be interviewed, then your response rate is still 60 percent. It would be inaccurate in this instance for telephone surveyors to report a response rate of 90 percent (180 out of 200). Ninety percent is really a "cooperation rate," not a response rate. You should consider all 300 patients in the denominator when computing the response rate.

Figure 8.2 provides a brief summary of the arguments for and against using three methods of data collection. All things considered, it is our recommendation that mailing surveys is the recommended method of data collection. Mailed questionnaires with an appropriate follow-up can obtain a 50 percent response rate or better with minimum expense, and without the interviewer bias typical of telephone surveys. In order to achieve this response rate, however, you

In Favor	Against
Mail Surveys	
• Inexpensive	• Slower Turnaround
• No Interviewer Bias	• Possible Low Response Rate
• Can Be Anonymous	
Phone Surveys	
• Fast Turnaround	• Expensive
• Personal	• Interviewer Bias
	• Interviewer Skill
	• Not Anonymous
	• Confusion of Cooperation Rate with Response Rate
Personally Distribute Questionnaires On Site (in Hospital or Office)	
• Inexpensive	• Not Anonymous
	• Leads to Positive Response Bias

FIGURE 8.2. Selecting the appropriate data collection method.

should have (1) a brief questionnaire (15 minutes or less) with an aesthetically appealing format, (2) an appropriate cover letter from the CEO, (3) a prepaid postage return envelope, and (4) at least one effort to follow-up on the original mailing either by mail or phone.

Report Format

If survey results are to influence decision making, they must be communicated in an appropriate report format. If you are displaying data from an enumerative study, an effective format should have several important components. First, provide comparative reference or benchmark data to allow the reader to see the data in context. Both internal comparisons (between nursing units, types of patients, previous surveys, and so forth) and external comparisons (with data from similar patients at other similar healthcare facilities) are valuable. Second, provide guidelines for interpreting the data so that the reader knows whether the observed differences are statistically significant and/or organizationally important. Finally, provide graphs of key findings in order to make tabular data more meaningful.

For example, Figure 8.3 is a sample report page from an enumerative study of inpatients. It displays graphs for three scales: medical outcome, physician care, and nursing care. First, notice that the graphs compare the results for the last four quarterly reports so that a manager can observe changes within the institution over time. Second, the report shows the mean, standard deviation, and range of scores for other similar hospitals with which the client hospital is being compared. These statistics allow the reader to determine how significant the difference between the hospital mean and the norm score actually is. Figure 8.3 also gives an example of a pie chart that enables the client hospital to visualize its own patient ratings of overall quality of care in comparison with the average scores of other hospitals.

On the other hand, if one is conducting an analytic study, then it is important to choose a control chart that is appropriate for the type of data obtained (i.e., variables or attribute data). For example, Figure 8.4 displays the scores from the physician subscale for eight consecutive quarters using an XmR chart. These data show that the average scale score for the last eight periods was 89.9 with an upper control limit of 92.5 and a lower control limit of 87.3. This chart shows that although the process has been in control for the past 2 years, all eight quarters are below the norm of other hospitals (91.15, which is provided on the top of Graph 5 in Figure 8.3). Therefore, when a process displays only common-cause variation, as it does in Figure 8.4, it can still present an opportunity for improvement.

Benchmark Data

Benchmark or comparative reference data help to place your facility's data into context. In Figure 8.3, the reader is able to see that the physician care subscale score for the current report is 90.37. If this was all the reader knew, it would be difficult to judge whether the process is improving or getting worse. By presenting the find-

MEMORIAL HOSPITAL
GROUP IS ALL PATIENTS
COMPARED TO NATIONAL NORM
CURRENT REPORT PERIOD IS:
APRIL – JUNE 1993
CLINICAL CARE
ALL PATIENTS
MEAN OF OTHER HOSPITALS
RANGE OF OTHER HOSPITALS
GRAPH 4:
MEDICAL OUTCOME SUBSCALE
NORM MEAN : 89.84
NORM S.D. : 2.73
SCALE SCORE
85.05
88.49
87.97
86.75
3 RPT. AGO
2 RPT. AGO
LAST RPT.
CURR. RPT.
GRAPH 5:
PHYSICIAN CARE SUBSCALE
NORM MEAN : 91.15
NORM S.D. : 2.00
90.21
90.27
88.74
90.37
GRAPH 6:
NURSING CARE SUBSCALE
NORM MEAN : 90.42
NORM S.D. : 3.11
88.10
89.80
90.93
90.75
GRAPH 7:
HOW WOULD YOU RATE THE OVERALL QUALITY OF CARE RECEIVED?
EXCELLENT 62%
FAIR/POOR 4%
GOOD 34%
OTHER HOSPITALS:
EXCELLENT 60%
GOOD 34%
FAIR/POOR 6%
PARKSIDE ASSOCIATES, INC.
INPATIENT QUALITY OF CARE MONITOR

FIGURE 8.3. Sample report page from enumerative study of inpatients.

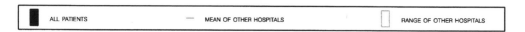

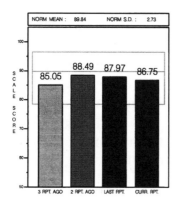

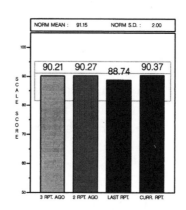

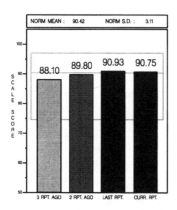

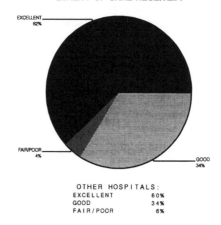

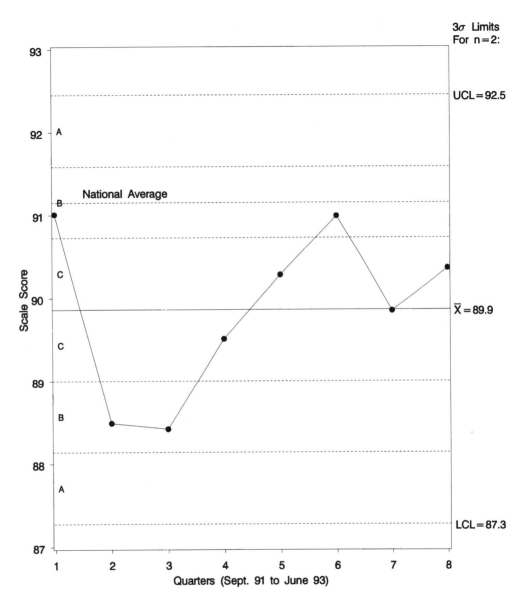

FIGURE 8.4. Physician care subscales for eight quarters (XmR chart).

ings for the previous three quarters (an internal benchmark), the reader can see that the results are fairly stable over the past year. On the other hand, using data from other similar hospitals as an external benchmark, the reader can also see that the scale scores are consistently below the average of other similar hospitals (referred to as the "norm"). This finding is even more forcefully presented in Figure 8.4 in the XmR control chart, where the average for the physician care subscale (89.9) is observed to be below the national average of 91.15 for eight consecutive quarters. The use of these internal and external benchmarks help to identify physician care as an opportunity for improvement.

The next step in improving the process (i.e., physician care in this example) would be to turn to a table listing the questions that compose the physician care scale and identify the specific aspects of physician care that need to be improved. For example, such a table (not presented here) might reveal that the patients were pleased with the overall courtesy and interpersonal skills of the physician, but were disappointed with the clarity of the explanation of diagnosis and treatment, or with the lack of clear discharge instructions.

External benchmark data are the most difficult to obtain. To make appropriate comparisons, data must be obtained using the same valid and reliable instrument, from similar patients at similar hospitals, with a representative response rate. Some research firms offer hospitals external benchmark data that are highly questionable because some or all of these requirements are missing. As individual hospitals join together to form large systems, however, the potential for consistent measurement of patient satisfaction will be enhanced.

Evaluating the Effectiveness of Interventions

Using surveys as enumerative studies, you can measure the voice of the customer both before and after an intervention to see whether or not the intervention had an effect (see Figure 8.1). The means of statistically analyzing the observed differences is discussed in other texts (Hayes, 1992).

Control charts plotting survey data can also be used to evaluate the effectiveness of interventions. In Figure 8.4, if you had made an intervention at the beginning of year 2 (between quarters 4 and 5) to improve the items on the physician care subscale, the control chart would demonstrate that this effort had not been very successful. No special cause was observed during the last four survey periods, and all of the eight quarters are still below the outside norm of 91.15.

On the other hand, it is important to recall that it usually requires 16 to 25 data points to obtain truly reliable control limits. Until one has at least 16 data points, it is better to refer to the upper and lower control limits as "trial limits." This is one of the reasons why survey research conducted on a quarterly schedule is best used as an enumerative study rather than an analytic study. Healthcare facilities that wish to use patient survey data for analytic studies should collect these data on a weekly or monthly schedule, so that they can obtain 16 to 25 data points in a more timely fashion. However, whether a facility is conducting surveys on a quarterly or monthly schedule, adequate attention always should be given to the reliability and validity of the questionnaire, the appropriateness of the sampling methodology, and the representatives of the response rate.

Summary

Under certain conditions, surveys can be used to conduct an analytic study to measure the voice of the process. However, given the time and resources required to obtain sufficient valid and reliable data, surveys in healthcare facilities are usually best used as enumerative studies to measure the voice of the customer and identify opportunities for improvement. Surveys, conducted less frequently but more carefully, can guide the focus of quality improvement efforts and measure the degree of improvement as perceived by patients.

However, whether you use surveys as enumerative or analytic studies, the quality of data will be enhanced by giving proper attention to reliability and validity, by appropriate sampling methods, by minimizing interviewer and response bias, and by appropriate graphing of results.

Appendix

Formulas for Calculating Control Limits

The formulas in this appendix cover the following types of charts:

- $\overline{X}$-R chart
- XmR chart
- p-Chart
- c-Chart
- u-Chart

The $\overline{X}$-R Chart

1. Decide on the number of observations (n) per subgroup.

2. Have 20 or more subgroups if possible.

3. Calculate the average ($\overline{X}$) and range (R) for each subgroup.

4. Calculate and plot:

   - $\overline{\overline{X}}$, *the average of a series of $\overline{X}$ values.*

   - $\overline{R}$, *the average of a series of ranges (R values).*

Average Chart Control Limits

- $$UCL = \overline{\overline{X}} + A_2 \overline{R}$$
  $$LCL = \overline{\overline{X}} - A_2 \overline{R}$$

Range Chart Control Limits

- $$UCL = D_4 \overline{R}$$
  $$LCL = D_3 \overline{R}$$

Where:

Subgroup size (n)	A_2	D_3	D_4
2	1.88	0	3.27
3	1.02	0	2.57
4	0.73	0	2.28
5	0.58	0	2.11
6	0.48	0	2.00
7	0.42	0.08	1.92
8	0.37	0.14	1.86
9	0.34	0.18	1.82
10	0.31	0.22	1.78

The XmR Chart

Formulas

1. *Process average* $= \overline{x}$

2. $\overline{x} = \dfrac{\sum x_i}{n}$

3. (a) *Compute the moving ranges (MRs)*
       adjacent data points.
    (b) *Then compute the mean range* $(\overline{R})$.

4. *Control limits* $= \overline{x} \pm 2.66\overline{R}$

The p–Chart

Formulas

1. *Process average* $= \overline{p}$

2. $\overline{p} = \dfrac{\text{number of defects}}{\text{total occurances}}$

3. $\hat{\sigma}^* = \sqrt{\dfrac{\overline{p}(1-\overline{p})}{n_i}}$

    Note: This value will vary as the units of observation vary.

4. Control limits $= \overline{p} \pm 3\sqrt{\dfrac{\overline{p}(1-\overline{p})}{n_i}}$

The c–Chart

Formulas

1. Process average $= \overline{c}$

2. $\overline{c} = \dfrac{\text{number of defects}}{\text{total observations}}$

3. $\hat{\sigma} = \sqrt{\bar{c}}$

4. Control limits $= \bar{c} \pm 3\sqrt{\bar{c}}$

The u–Chart

Formulas

1. Process average $= \bar{u}$

2. $\bar{u} = \dfrac{\text{number of defects for all subgroups}}{\text{total number of observations in all subgroups}}$

3. $\hat{\sigma}* = \sqrt{\dfrac{\bar{u}}{n_i \text{ (of each subgroup)}}}$

   Note: This value will vary as the subgroup size varies.

4. Control limits $= \bar{u} \pm 3\sqrt{\dfrac{\bar{u}}{n_1}}$

References

Austin, Charles. *Information Systems for Hospital Administration*. Health Administration Press, 1983.

Babbie, E. R. *The Practice of Social Research*. Belmont, CA: Wadsworth, 1989.

Berwick, Donald M. "Buckling Down to Change," A presentation to the Fifth Annual National Forum on Quality Improvement in Healthcare. Orlando, FL: December, 1993.

Blalock, Hubert M., *Social Statistics*. New York: McGraw-Hill, 1960.

Blumenthal, David. "Total Quality Management and Physicians Clinical Decisions," *Journal of the American Medical Association*, Vol. 269, No. 21, 1993, pp. 2775–2778.

Carey, Raymond G. and Seibert, Jerry H. "A Patient Survey System to Measure Quality Improvement," *Medical Care*, Vol. 31, No. 19, Sept. 1993.

Cronbach, L. "Coefficient Alpha and the Internal Structure of Tests," *Psychometrika*, 1951, pp. 16–297.

Deming, W. Edwards. "On a Classification of the Problems of Statistical Inference," *Journal of the American Statistical Association*, Vol. 37, No. 218, 1942, pp. 173–185.

Deming, W. Edwards. "On Probability as a Basis for Action," *The American Statistician*, Vol. 29, No. 4, 1975, pp. 146–152.

Deming, W. Edwards. *Out of the Crisis*. Cambridge: Massachusetts Institute of Technology, Center for Advanced Engineering Study, 1986.

Duncan, Acheson J. *Quality Control and Industrial Statistics*. Homewood, IL: Irwin, 1986.

Feigenbaum, A. V. *Total Quality Control*. New York: McGraw-Hill, 1988.

Gitlow, Howard, Gitlow, Shelly, Oppenheim, Alan, Oppenheim, Rosa. *Tools and Methods for the Improvement of Quality*. Homewood, IL: Irwin, 1989.

Harman, Harry H. *Modern Factor Analysis*. Chicago, IL: University of Chicago Press, 1976.

Hayes, Bob E. *Measuring Customer Satisfaction*. Milwaukee, WI: ASQC Quality Press, 1992.

Helmstadter, G. C. *Principles of Psychological Measurement*. New York: Appleton—Century—Crofts, 1964.

Hospital Research and Educational Trust. *Inventory of External Data Demands Placed on Hospitals*. Chicago: Quality Measurement and Management Project, Hospital Research and Educational Trust, 1990.

Ishikawa, Kaoru. *Guide to Quality Control*. New York: Quality Resources, 1989.

Lastrucci, Carlo L. *The Scientific Approach*. Cambridge: Schenkmon, 1967.

Montgomery, Douglas C., *Introduction to Statistical Quality Control Second Edition.* New York: John Wiley & Sons, 1991.

Nunnally, J. C. *Psychometric Theory.* New York: McGraw-Hill, 1967.

Patton, Michael Q. *How to Use Qualitative Methods in Evaluation.* Newbury Park, CA: Sage, 1987.

Plsek, Paul E. "Tutorial: Introduction to Control Charts," *Quality Management in Health Care,* Vol. 1, No. 1, 1992, pp. 65–74.

Plsek, Paul E., and Onnias, Arturo. *Quality Improvement Tools.* Wilton, CT: Juran Institute, Inc., 1989.

Pyzdek, Thomas. *Pyzdek's Guide to SPC—Volume One: Fundamentals.* Milwaukee: ASQC Quality Press, 1990.

Roberts, Lon. *Process Reengineering: The Key to Achieving Breakthrough Success.* Milwaukee: ASQC Quality Press, 1994.

Scholtes, Peter R. *The Team Handbook: How to Use Teams to Improve Quality.* Madison, WI: Joiner Associates, 1988.

Selltiz, Claire. *Research Methods in Social Relations.* New York: Holt, Rinehart and Winston, 1959.

Shewhart, Walter A. *Economic Control of Quality of Manufactured Product.* New York: Van Nostrand, 1931.

Sloan, Daniel M. *How to Lower Healthcare Costs by Improving Healthcare Quality.* Milwaukee: ASQC Quality Press, 1994.

Torki, Neviene. *The Link—Statistical Techniques—Process Improvement.* Melbourne, Australia: Imageset, 1992.

Western Electric Company. *Statistical Quality Control Handbook.* Indianapolis: AT&T Technologies Inc., 1984.

Wheeler, Donald J. *Understanding Variation: The Key to Managing Chaos.* Knoxville, TN: SPC Press, 1993.

Wheeler, Donald J. and Chambers, David S. *Understanding Statistical Process Control.* Knoxville, TN: SPC Press, 1992.

INDEX